Christian Couples Coping with Childlessness

American Society of Missiology Monograph Series

The ASM Monograph Series provides a forum for publishing quality dissertations and studies in the field of missiology. Collaborating with Pickwick Publications—a division of Wipf and Stock Publishers of Eugene, Oregon—the American Society of Missiology selects high quality dissertations and other monographic studies that offer research materials in mission studies for scholars, mission and church leaders, and the academic community at large. The ASM seeks scholarly work for publication in the Series that throws light on issues confronting Christian world mission in its cultural, social, historical, biblical, and theological dimensions.

Missiology is an academic field that brings together scholars whose professional training ranges from doctoral-level preparation in areas such as scripture, history and sociology of religions, anthropology, theology, international relations, interreligious interchange, mission history, inculturation, and church law. The American Society of Missiology, which sponsors this series, is an ecumenical body drawing members from Independent and Ecumenical Protestant, Catholic, Orthodox, and other traditions. Members of the ASM are united by their commitment to reflect on and do scholarly work relating to both mission history and the present-day mission of the church. The ASM Monograph Series aims to publish works of exceptional merit on specialized topics, with particular attention given to work by younger scholars, the dissemination and publication of which is difficult under the economic pressures of standard publishing models.

Persons seeking information about the ASM or the guidelines for having their dissertations considered for publication in the ASM Monograph Series should consult the Society's website—www.asmweb.org.

Members of the ASM Monograph Committee who approved this book are:

Paul Kollman
University of Notre Dame

Michael A. Rynkiewich
Asbury Theological Seminary

Judith Lingenfelter
Biola University

Christian Couples Coping with Childlessness

Narratives from Machame, Kilimanjaro

AULI VÄHÄKANGAS

American Society of Missiology
Monograph Series

4

☙PICKWICK *Publications* · Eugene, Oregon

CHRISTIAN COUPLES COPING WITH CHILDLESSNESS
Narratives from Machame, Kilimanjaro

American Society of Missiology Monograph Series 4

Copyright © 2009 Auli Vähäkangas. All rights reserved. No part of this publication may be reproduced or transmitted in any form, electronic or mechanical, or stored on any information storage and retrieval system without prior permission in writing from the publishers. For permissions write to Wipf & Stock Publishers, 199 W. 8th Avenue, Suite 3, Eugene OR 97401.

Pickwick Publications
A Division of Wipf and Stock Publishers
199 W. 8th Ave., Suite 3
Eugene, OR 97401

www.wipfandstock.com

ISBN: 978-1-60608-652-0

Cataloguing-In-Publication data:

Vähäkangas, Auli

    Christian couples coping with childlessness : narratives from Machame, Kilimanjaro / Auli Vähäkangas

    viii + 186 p. ; 23 cm. Includes bibliographical references and index.

    American Society of Missiology Monograph Series 4

    ISBN: 978-1-60608-652-0

    1. Infertility—Africa. 2. Infertility—Religious aspects. I. Title. II. Series.

RC889 V25 2009

Manufactured in the United States of America

Books published in the American Society of Missiology Scholarly monograph series are chosen on the basis of their academic quality as responsible contributions to debate and dialogue about issues in mission studies. The opinions expressed in the book are those of the authors and are not represented to be those of the American Society of Missiology or its members.

Contents

Preface / vii

List of Illustrations / viii

Introduction / 1

1. Research Procedure / 23
2. Narrative of a Committed Union / 56
3. Narrative of Desertion / 71
4. Two Narratives of Polygyny / 94
5. Life of Childless Couples in Machame / 111
6. Sense of Coherence as Wholeness / 149

Conclusion / 158

Appendices:
    A: Sample Interview Questions / 163
    B: Direct Quotations in Swahili / 164

Glossary / 173

Bibliography / 175

Index / 185

Preface

DURING MY RESEARCH, I have been privileged to meet many people in the Northern Diocese of the Evangelical Lutheran Church in Tanzania. I would like to express my special thanks to all of them. I would like to remind them, however, that they will not find authentic life stories of their friends and neighbors in this study.

The advice of the late professor Cuthbert Omari to properly focus my field research was valuable in the planning stage. My warmest appreciation goes to my advisor, Professor Eila Helander, for her wise supervision and cheery encouragement. Professor Arvi Hurskainen has gifted me with the knowledge of language as well as culture, and has examined my text during the final process of its approval as a doctoral dissertation.

Päivi Hasu, whom I met while she was conducting her own field research among the Chagga of Kilimanjaro in the 1990s, has contributed much more to my dissertation than she can believe. Discussions with her in different parts of the globe—London, Finland, Tanzania—have contributed much to my understanding of the Chagga culture. She has also tirelessly read and commented on various manuscripts.

One important community that has given me both constructive criticism and faithful support has been the Tanzania Theological Colloquium group. My Tanzanian colleagues' criticism of my interpretations has aided me in correcting some of them and in giving stronger supporting evidence for others.

Marvin Kananen and Helen Davico have adeptly revised my English, and I want to thank them for this great work. Professor Ishmael Mbise checked the language of the Swahili quotations. If there are any mistakes or stylistic faults, they are certainly due to my lack of attention.

My sincere gratitude goes to my beloved husband Mika and to our three daughters Irinja, Eliisa, and Pauliina, who had to cope with my heavy workload. Mika, a systematic theologian, challenged my interpretations during our daily walks in the neighboring coffee farm.

My name giver, Irinja, turned ten while I was finalizing this research project. This ten-year period has taught me a lot about my identity in the African community, as well as about the identity construction of Christian couples in Machame. The research process has been much more than just an academic exercise; it has been part of my own life story.

Illustrations

Table 1	Interviewees in two study parishes
Table 2	Distribution of Age
Table 3	Place of Birth
Table 4	Code Categories Used in Atlas-ti© Program
Table 5	Interviews Used to Construct Model Narratives
Table 6	The Differences between Two Polygynous Marriages
Table 7	Comparison of the Lives of Three Second Wives
Table 8	Construction of Male Identity of Men of Model Narratives
Table 9	Construction of Female Identity of Four Childless Wives
Table 10	Insults about Childless Wife
Table 11	Inner and Outer Resources of Childless Individuals
Table 12	Individual and Joint Coping Strategies

Introduction

Why Don't You Have a Child Yet?

I unexpectedly encountered the issue of childlessness in Tanzania shortly after my arrival in 1990. I was frequently asked: "How long have you been married? Why don't you have a child yet?" The implication of the latter question was that there was something wrong with me, since I was married, in my twenties, and still childless. Those questions and their implications followed me constantly. They tainted my time in Tanzania.

Three years later when back in Tanzania, our first child was born. Her presence in my life changed my status in Tanzanian society. No longer was I looked upon as being abnormal, immoral, cursed, or whatever the full implication of their question might have been, but I was then known as Mama Irinja. I was no longer called by my own name but by the name of my firstborn.

It was in the transition of my social status in Tanzania that I began to see the incredible social pressure that is put on women who are childless. It is this aspect of society I wish to address in this study—the problems and the pains of childlessness as seen in two specific Christian communities in the Kilimanjaro region of Tanzania.

Childlessness is not only a problem for an individual woman, but also a concern of the whole community. The number of infertile women in Tanzania, especially in the northern region, is not very high when compared to international figures. In 1996 the percentage of childless women was 4 percent in urban areas and just two percent in rural areas. Included in this data are women who have been married seven years or more and remain without children. Larsen and Raggers note that primary infertility in urban areas is higher in Tanzania than in most of the countries analyzed.[1] The fact that Western infertility cures are often unavailable further complicates the life of infertile couples. Many infertile women will stay infertile for the rest of their lives. Infertility is not a primary concern for national health policy. The main interest of

---

1. Larsen and Raggers, "Levels and Trends," 39–40, 46.

Tanzanian health policies is limiting fertility and teaching family planning, not helping those who have problems bearing children—even though children are highly regarded in the culture.

Children have high economic and non-economic value in Tanzania. Their economic role in a country without a functioning social security system is very important. Children are the financial security of their parents and an important labor force.[2] The non-economic value of children corresponds to the psychic satisfaction parents derive from them. Through children individuals gain a respected status in the community—people are only defined as adults after they become parents. The desire for children also includes the aspects of seeking immortality and improving quality of life. Immortality through procreation is an important traditional value in various ethnic societies of Tanzania. The quality of life is expected to come from the joy children bring into a family. Because both aspects of the value attached to children are important in Tanzania, the problem of childlessness is an even deeper personal and communal problem than in Western countries.[3] Although the value of children in an urban setting differs from that in a rural agrarian community, the desire to have children has not declined even in urban communities of Tanzania.

Infertility can lead to stigma. Perhaps unfairly, it is women who are the most stigmatized in Tanzania because of infertility, but it is also a serious problem for men.[4] Not having children is considered deviant behavior for both women and men. Children continue to be important for strengthening the marital and kinship ties in a changing society. The desire to have children has not decreased in the process of social change and urbanization,[5] a dynamic that will be discussed below.

The Crisis of Marriage in a Changing Society

Social, Political, and Religious Changes in Tanzania

In the past ten years Tanzania has experienced profound political, economic, and social changes. The change from a one-party system to a multiparty system and the rapid economical and social changes have deeply influenced its society. Urbanization is rampant in various centers around the country. Tanzania is living in a time of transition from rural agrarian

---

2. Howard and Millard, *Hunger and Shame*, 142.
3. Mgalla and Boerma, "Discourse of Infertility," 196; Gijsels et. al., "'No Child Send,'" 209–11.
4. Gijsels et. al., "'No Child Send,'" 214–15, 219.
5. Kanyongo-Male and Onyango, *Sociology*, 105.

community to urban market economy.⁶ At the moment, both traditional agrarian communities and large urban cities are found in the same country. Most of the young people migrate to towns from rural villages. In towns they face a new set of values and a completely new way of life.

Religious changes have also been rapid. In the beginning of 1990s the national policy of Tanzania toward new religious groups became more open. Until recently, in northern Tanzania the historical churches, mainly the Lutheran and Roman Catholic churches, had dominated. Changes in the religious environment have greatly influenced families in Tanzania, especially in the urban areas. Family life in villages is still closer to the traditional form in which all members of a household—and often a whole village—belong to the same denomination. The urban situation is more pluralistic, where the members of one household often belong to various religious groups. People often still belong to official churches but attend services elsewhere where they find more meaningful beliefs and practices.

The rapid social shifts have changed the structure of Tanzanian society. The breakdown of traditional social structures has left some people isolated. In a traditional community there is always somebody older who can give advice and guidance on how to handle difficult situations,⁷ but the changing structures have led to the growth of individualism. The family is not as strong a source of support and control as it used to be in traditional communities.⁸

The loosening of communal control has led to an increase of venereal diseases and contributed to the rapid spread of Human Immunodeficiency Virus (HIV) and Acquired Immune Deficiency Syndrome (AIDS) in many parts of Tanzania. Infections from sexually transmitted diseases (STDs) have been found to be the major cause of infertility in sub-Saharan Africa.⁹ Research has shown that infertility may also be a risk factor for HIV and STDs.¹⁰ The spread of HIV/AIDS has greatly influenced the life of most families in Kilimanjaro. Many youngsters who work in towns become infected there. In all villages in Kilimanjaro there are AIDS patients to be cared for, and funerals have become the most common function in the Lutheran parishes there.

These social, political, economic, and religious changes in Tanzania have led to a growing number of personal identities. Identities shift in

---

6. Bahemuka and Brockington, preface to *East Africa*, xv.
7. Domingues, *Christ Our Healer*, 103–4.
8. Peil and Oyeneye, *Consensus, Conflict and Change*, 169.
9. Larsen and Raggers, "Levels and Trends," 26.
10. Gijsels et. al., "'No Child Send,'" 219.

response to situational contexts. When people speak Swahili they call up their national identity as Tanzanian citizens. When they use their ethnic language they emphasize their ethnic and local identity. Similarly, religious identity might change depending on the situation; while visiting the villages people identify themselves with the historical churches where their families have belonged for generations, but when in the urban situation their religious identity might not be that strong or it might shift to a different denomination.[11] Education has also been a tool of social change in many parts of Tanzania. Professor Lawuo has criticized the system of church schools, which, he argues, have destroyed ethnic identities and strengthened imported religious identities.[12] This situation of the family and shifting identities in a changing society is discussed in more detail in the following section.

Chagga Family in a Changing Society

The setting of this study is in northern Tanzania, in the Machame cultural area of Chaggaland. Machame is located in western Kilimanjaro. It used to be an independent kingdom during German and British colonialism, whereas now it is not a separate administrative unit but forms a part of the Hai district of the Kilimanjaro region. Most of the inhabitants in this area share a common Chagga ethnic background. One patriclan forms localized clusters of patrilineal kinsmen. In indigenous Chaggaland, the patriclan is a group of people who share the same ancestry and are, therefore, related by blood.[13] Usually one patriclan is identified by a common name. In the Machame area the most common family names are Swai, Nkya, and Shoo. Each clan is related to several others through marriages. The whole Chagga society is an interconnected web in which everyone feels closely related to everyone else. The community that has an interest in a family's bearing of children is thus broad. In Kilimanjaro, clan members are in close connection with each other, and the community is understood to include the dead and those who are yet to be born into a clan.

In transitional society, the different cultural categories work side by side. In contemporary Kilimanjaro, three different systems of practice can be classified: *kienyeji* (traditional), *kikristo* (Christian), and *kisasa* (modern).[14] *Kienyeji* refers to the Chagga traditions. Some of these remain

---

11. See Tessler et al., *Tradition and Identity*, 93, 97.
12. Lawuo, *Education and Social Change*, 129–41.
13. Mosha, *Heartbeat*, 146; Moore, "Chagga of Kilimanjaro," 32.
14. Comaroff and Comaroff, *Christianity, Colonialism*, 212; Hasu, *Desire and Death*, 41–42.

now only as oral history, but others are still followed. *Kikristo* refers to imported Christian beliefs and practices, especially the teachings of the early missionaries—therefore, it does not refer directly to the teachings of the Lutheran church in the Kilimanjaro area. *Kisasa* is used in this research to denote those cultural practices and beliefs that result from education, modernization, and urbanization in Kilimanjaro. These historically motivated cultural categories help people find their way in the changing society, but they also lead to a tension between different frames of reference.

The Chagga construct their personal and social identities on the cultural categories discussed above. Usually one individual compiles his/her personal identity from at least two of these categories. The same individual can change his/her approach during the course of life. Older people tend to rely more on *kienyeji*, while the younger, urban Chagga rely more on *kisasa*. The situation is, however, much more complicated than just age or rural-urban differences, as will be analyzed later in this research.

Adding to the cultural category tensions, labor migration influences the life of the Chagga families. Many men migrate into towns and cities around Tanzania, leaving their wives in Kilimanjaro. Migration has increased both geographical separation and marital separation. The traditional gender roles are also changing through migration. The women who are left at the mountain have to take care of all household duties and make decisions within the family that were traditionally made by the men. The single parent situation has increased the freedom of women; however, at the same time, marital situations have become more unstable than in the traditional society.

In recent years there seems to be a growing trend not to leave the family behind. More often entire Chagga families migrate to towns inside and outside the Kilimanjaro region. Urbanization has decreased the need for larger family units because in towns there is not room for as many relatives to live with a family as in the rural community. However, even in the urban communities the African family is usually larger than the Western nuclear family.

Christian Marriage in the Northern Diocese

This study is carried out in the Northern Diocese of the Evangelical Lutheran Church in Tanzania (ELCT). The Northern Diocese is one of the oldest and, in previous years, one of the most financially well-off and stable of the twenty Lutheran dioceses in Tanzania. The Northern Diocese and its parishes follow the guidelines of the constitution of the diocese and also the constitution of the whole ELCT. Lutherans originating from the Northern Diocese area are nowadays influential in many other dioceses of the ELCT, especially in the Eastern and Coastal Diocese (Dar es Salaam) and in the East of Lake Victoria Diocese (Mwanza). Intensive labor migration has spread the influence of Chagga Christians across the whole country, into each area of the ELCT.

The Kilimanjaro area is strongly Christian. Lutheran and Catholic Christians make up the majority of the inhabitants in rural Kilimanjaro. In more urban centers, Islam and different types of Pentecostal churches also have a significant number of followers. In the Kilimanjaro area, there are very few people who are officially still followers of African traditional religions. However, many Catholic and Lutheran Christians also follow some of the practices and beliefs of the traditional religions.

Christian marriage in this study denotes the marriage between two Christians, namely, people who belong to the Christian church and identify themselves with it. Lutheran theology includes marriage as part of a secular sphere and does not make a theological distinction between a Christian and a secular marriage. To Lutheran Christians in Tanzania, however, there is a difference. In common discussions on marriage, people seem to distinguish between a Christian marriage, which in their understanding points to a church wedding and restrictions against cohabitation, and a purely secular marriage.

The constitution of the Northern Diocese uses the term "marriage of a Christian."[15] The use of the singular is noticeable in this case; in marriage there are two people involved. The logic behind it seems to be that the man is counted to be the Christian who marries, while the woman is the one who is being married. The man has the active role in a Chagga marriage. Swahili terminology also expresses this active role; a man is the one who marries, a woman gets married. Patriarchal traditions on family life and roles of spouses continue to influence the life of Chagga Christians in the contemporary society.

The constitution gives additional requirements for a marriage in the Northern Diocese. The marriage age follows the Marriage Act regulations of year 1971.[16] Both the man and the woman have to be full members of the Lutheran church, which means that they have to be baptized and confirmed in the church and not under church discipline.[17] In a case where

---

15. ELCT, Constitution 1986, 68.

16. Westerlund, "Marriage and Religion," 99; Bahendwa, *Christian Religious Education*, 273.

17. ELCT, Constitution 1986, 68.

one of the engaged persons is a member of another Protestant denomination, there can still be a church wedding. In the constitution there is an expressed wish for Lutheran Christians not to marry Roman Catholics because children born into such a union would probably be baptized into the Roman Catholic faith. In cases where one is a follower of a non-Christian community, the marriage cannot be officiated in the church. This type of marriage can later be blessed in the church if the non-Christian spouse is baptized. If a Christian is under church discipline, he or she has to repent and welcomed back into the participation of Eucharist before the marriage can be blessed in the parish.[18]

The Northern Diocese follows a tradition derived from Matthew 5:9 requiring a marriage to have two sponsors who must be adult Christians who live in a proper Christian marriage themselves and are mentally fit.[19] Usually these sponsors are a married couple. In the practice of the Northern Diocese, these sponsors are the first ones to counsel the young couple if there are any problems in the marriage. There is some debate as to how these sponsors should be chosen. At the moment, the practice is that the couple chooses their close friends to be sponsors if they meet the requirements of the constitution. Older people and church workers protest that these sponsors are not always well-equipped to counsel a Christian marriage in contemporary society.

The Northern Diocese does not accept divorce. The reason given in the constitution is that if God has united a couple, human beings should not separate them.[20] In practice, however, there are divorces in Kilimanjaro. Many of them are merely long-term separations, while other couples go to a civil court to have their marriage dissolved.[21]

The Catholic Church uses the term "Christian marriage" to stress the sacramental nature of marriage. This sacramental understanding of a marriage differs from that of Lutheran definition of marriage, even though the common understanding of a Christian marriage in Kilimanjaro seems not to differ much between Lutheran and Roman Catholic Christians. In the understanding of the Catholic Church, marriage cannot be dissolved except in a few special cases such as the madness of a spouse. In these cases the pope himself has to give permission for a divorce. The practice of the Northern Diocese not to accept divorce comes, interestingly, very close to the Roman Catholic sacramental nature of marriage.

18. Ibid., 69–70.
19. Ibid., 71.
20. Ibid., 73.
21. Westerlund, "Marriage and Religion," 100.

This is perhaps because pietistic teachings have influenced the understanding of Christian marriage among Lutherans in Tanzania. The stress on individualism, important to Pietism, contradicts the communal values of Chagga society. Missionaries introduced Christian marriage into parishes and often did not understand the cultural values behind an indigenous marriage. For example, an important part of the traditional marriage arrangements in Kilimanjaro was that a marriage was an affair of the whole community. Both families were involved and were responsible for preparing the young couple for marriage. The beginning of marriage was understood to be a process that included many functions and rituals, not merely one celebration.[22]

The questions of marriage and family remain a central pastoral theme in the Lutheran church in Tanzania, especially in the Northern Diocese. The pandemia of HIV/AIDS has influenced the discourse on family values. Pastors have to face many marital problems almost daily in their work in the local parishes. Some of these problems include wife beating, polygyny, deserting of wives, and children born out of wedlock. Many of these problems actually result from childlessness—especially lack of sons—in the marriage. It seems that pastors do not have enough tools to deal with these problems. The Northern Diocese uses the practice of church discipline in order to direct those who act against the norms of the church. In specific terms of the constitution of the Northern Diocese, nobody is actually put under church discipline; it is the individual Christian who separates herself or himself from the parish when acting against its laws.[23] In ordinary language, people still assume that somebody is put under church discipline and this is how the practice actually works. However, it seems that time has weakened the practice of church discipline.

In the Marriage Act of 1971, the Republic of Tanzania clearly states that all marriages, whether Christian, Muslim, or customary, are valid. Christian marriage, according to Tanzanian law, cannot be made polygynous.[24] Many Christians begin with "shortcut marriages," which they later on seek to have blessed in the church. Many couples do not fulfill the requirements to be married in the church, often because they have cohabited first, had a child before marriage, or lacked the financial resources to organize a church wedding. It seems that most marriage functions in the contemporary Lutheran parishes are blessings of an existing civil marriage,

---

22. Moore, "Chagga of Kilimanjaro," 36.
23. ELCT, Constitution 1986, 77.
24. Westerlund, "Marriage and Religion," 99.

and that formal church weddings actually constitute only a very small percentage of the marriage functions.[25]

Many Christians are confused about the Christian teachings on marriage, which seem to stress the importance of a church wedding, while at the same time the number of church weddings is relatively small. Contradicting influences, like the pietistic Lutheran teachings versus the Chagga traditions, have left people in a difficult situation. Parishioners seem to define a Christian marriage as one inaugurated with fancy church wedding, whereas the non-Christian "shortcut marriage"—as well as cohabitation—appears to be more common in the everyday world.

My observations on the current marital situation evoked my interest to find out what had been previously studied in various fields in connection to marriage and infertility. I found that Chagga marriage and family patterns have been studied to some extent, the findings of which I review in the following section. The research on Chagga traditions regarding fertility and patriarchy will be discussed first, after which the central topics of recent anthropological gender research in Kilimanjaro area will be analyzed. Multidisciplinary studies on infertility are discussed next, followed by a review of the theological discussion about the value of children in Christian marriage in Africa.

Previous Research

Fertility and Patriarchy in Chagga Ethnographies

The Chagga ethnic group has been studied extensively by both expatriates and the Chagga themselves. The large quantity of ethnographic material produced has provided valuable background information for planning the field research for this study. Among these early documentations is a note on the burial of a childless woman. She is not buried properly; her body is thrown in the bush together with all of her belongings.[26] The account of burial practices shows how childlessness influenced the whole community in the Chagga history. Infertility is analyzed from the communal point of view, revealing the importance of the search for the reason behind barrenness. After reading the history of the Chagga, I wanted to find out what the consequences of childlessness in the modern Chagga community are.

The marriage traditions and reasons for divorce have also been analyzed in Chagga ethnographies. Divorce because of barrenness was possible only after trying many different types of medicines and after offering

25. Pietilä, *Gossip, Markets and Gender*, 214; Hasu, *Desire and Death*, 536.
26. Gutmann, "Totenreich," 200; Dundas, *Kilimanjaro*, 181.

many sacrifices to the ancestors. Only male children were counted when dealing with the reasons a wife could be deserted. If a woman had only female children she was regarded as if she did not have any children. If the reason for divorce was barrenness, the husband did not have to pay the bride wealth back, but rather, only one cow, which was considered the salary for the work the woman had done in her husband's farm.[27]

Fertility was considered comparable with the concept of immortality in traditional Chagga society. Children were needed both for the purpose of remembrance and in order that they could perform the appropriate sacrifices needed for their parents to die peacefully. The Chagga community consists of more than those living at the moment; it includes departed ancestors.[28] Immortality is an important theme in the ethnographies. I wanted to find out whether this has affected the life of Christian couples in the contemporary situation. A sterility case in a local court, involving accusations of witchcraft between the wives of two brothers, is also documented in the Chagga ethnographies. This sterility case, even though it happened in eastern Kilimanjaro more than fifty years ago, gives an important insight into the communal aspect of infertility. Moore's analysis includes the impact of the case to the whole lineage and the role that the church played in it.[29]

The Chagga ethnographies describe a patrilineal society in the Kilimanjaro area. Chagga society traces its lineage to the father, who is the head of the family. As the head, the father has authority over his children and his wife/wives. This valuable ethnographical material has documented the Chagga customs and beliefs in such a way that it is difficult to find another ethnic group that has been so carefully studied. These ethnographies include some references to infertility, but concentrate mainly on describing certain rituals that were done in order to find the cause of infertility or to increase fertility.

The ethnographical data is old and does not deal with the problem of childlessness in the contemporary Chagga society. It does reveal, however, the other important topics connected to childlessness in Chagga community: burial and the rituals connected to it, the question of immortality, and the effects of childlessness within marriage. This ethnographic material gave me a good background of information from which to perform in-depth analysis of contemporary Chagga society.

---

27. Gutmann, *Frau bei den Wadschagga*, 31; Marealle, *Maisha ya Mchagga*, 48–49.
28. Moore, "Secret of the Men," 358; 1977, 47; Gutmann, *Frau bei den Wadschagga*, 1.
29. Moore, *Social Facts*, 259–62.

Anthropological Gender Research in Kilimanjaro

Recent anthropological research concentrates on the lives of young people during the time of HIV/AIDS. These studies concentrate on the sexual roles and behavior of people in Northern Tanzania in the 1990s. I begin here with an overview of these studies, which contributed some insights to my own study, and conclude with those which come closer to my own topic.

Chagga people see themselves as people of civilization, contrary to some other ethnic groups who the Chagga, according to Tuulikki Pietilä's findings, describe as people of the bush. This identity of being modern and open to new inventions is central for the Chagga of Kilimanjaro. Pietilä, who focused on gossip as a way to search for knowledge in Kilimanjaro, does discuss female moral values, but she does not deal much with the importance of children to the female identity. She analyzes the life of unmarried women in the Chagga society, but does not evaluate the difference between those unmarried women who have children and those who do not.[30]

The influence of modernization and education on traditional Chagga family values, especially on the gender roles in family, has been studied by Amy Stambach.[31] She explores how collective ideas about what is modern and traditional, in particular how age and gender are formulated in multiple ways, and how these ideas emerge in connection with people's understandings of schooling.[32] Many high school girls, in reply to her questions, said they would like to continue their studies and were not interested in getting married and staying at home. When Stambach came back to the same area in Machame five years later and reinterviewed these former schoolgirls, she found that most of them were married and had children. Additionally, most had not continued their education after secondary school. Their initial wishes had not come true.[33] Stambach's research reveals that modernization has not really changed the life of women in Kilimanjaro; the role expectations for them remain similar to that of the traditional society. This means, primarily, that a woman is supposed to become a mother. Motherhood seems to be central to the female role even in the case of the younger Chagga generation, even among the more educated girls.

From her studies in the 1990s Päivi Hasu reveals interesting case studies on sexual relations and their influence on the institution of mar-

---

30. Pietilä, *Gossip, Markets and Gender*, 48–72, 138–62, 214–19.
31. Stambach, *Lessons*.
32. Ibid., 10.
33. Ibid., 61–64.

riage in the Mwika area in eastern Kilimanjaro. Hasu discusses Christian moral discourse during the time of HIV/AIDS.[34] Hasu's in-depth analysis of the Chagga rituals and practices, and their input into the life of the modern Chagga in a rural village, give information on both the old traditions and the modern situation. The majority of people in the Mwika area are Lutherans. Hasu did not concentrate directly on the church community, but her findings do reveal the values and practices of Lutherans in the area in which she conducted her study.

Philip Setel and his Tanzanian colleagues have studied the value of fertility and its influence on the marriage agreement. They found, in their study in an urban ward of Moshi town, that the need to have children is one reason to delay the sealing of a marriage in a church.[35] They do not, however, deal with the pastoral side of the problem of infertility. As a team consisting of an anthropologist and health workers, their task was not to deal with the theology of marriage, leaving the pastoral side to be dealt with by theological research, such as in the present study.

All these recent anthropological studies have been conducted either at a village level or in other secular contexts such as schools. Hasu did pay attention to the importance of church community in Kilimanjaro, but the others payed little attention to it. Stambach is the only one who did her study in the Machame area of western Kilimanjaro. Hasu and Pietilä conducted their research in east Kilimanjaro, whereas Setel and his colleagues collected their data in Moshi town, which is located in central Kilimanjaro. My own study, which is conducted in two Christian communities in western Kilimanjaro, considers the Christian influence on family life in this less studied region.

Multidisciplinary Studies on Infertility

Infertility has been studied in various fields, and many different methods have been used. In this section I refer to those studies, divided into four groups, that most gave me insight during the process of my own study. The first group is mainly quantitative population studies on fertility in sub-Saharan Africa. They provided me with statistics of infertility and with some biological reasons for infertility. They did not, however, contribute much to the understanding of the life of an infertile couple in Kilimanjaro. The second group consists of psychosocial studies on infertile couples from different contexts. These psychosocial studies, which, in

---

34. Hasu, *Desire and Death*, 23, 243–91.
35. Setel el al., "Men's perspectives," 12.

spite of having been done mainly in Western setting, gave some insight into the life of infertile couples in Africa. The third group consists of case studies of infertile women in Egypt and India. These case studies served as a methodological guide and a good comparison to my somewhat similar life story data, even though the context of the current study differs from Egypt and India. The fourth and the most valuable group consists of multidisciplinary qualitative studies on the impact of fertility and infertility in the life of women and men in different African societies.

Population studies focus on infertility in Africa mainly using a quantitative approach. Roushdi A. Henin's findings reveal that infertility and sub-fertility are associated with the degree of economic and social development and with different marital habits. What is interesting in Henin's study is that he describes the northeast Highlands of Tanzania as an economically prosperous area with high fertility rates and low childlessness rates. He found that the childlessness rate is low there because of better nutrition and lower sickness rates. As an example, he mentions that in the Highlands malaria is very rare, whereas in many other parts of Tanzania where malaria is more common there is a corresponding higher infertility rate.[36] In particular, his findings that the climate in Kilimanjaro and the more nutritious diet of the Chagga have decreased the problem of childlessness are helpful for my research. Malaria is currently climbing into areas of higher altitude because of climatic changes in the region. These findings raise important questions: Is the infertility rate still low compared to other parts of Tanzania? What factors contribute to the infertility rate other than nutrition and climate as found by Henin?

Population studies written during the time of *Ujamaa* socialism connect economic production and human reproduction together. Ulla Vuorela expanded the historical materialist theory of the modes of production in her analysis of human reproduction. The focus of her study was the nature of the social relations of production, the basis of subsistence, and the social relations of human reproduction.[37] She concentrates more on production than on reproduction, which may be due to the fact that her study was done during the financially difficult times in Tanzania before the open market economy was introduced in the late 1980s. Vuorela's research context was a traditional village, a small Kwere village close to Chalinze, where further descriptions of life and different case studies are central. As the Kwere are matrilineal people of coastal Tanzania, comparison with Vuorela's findings enabled me to see the strong patrilineal nature of the

36. Henin "Fertility," 12.
37. Vuorela, *Women's Question*, 4–8.

Chagga society. Among the Kwere, fertility is central to women because they continue the lineage. Among the Chagga, continuation follows the paternal lineage. The value of reproduction among the Chagga is thus central to both male and female identity, in comparison to the Kwere community where reproduction is mainly a female concern.

Students of the University of Dar es Salaam have studied infertility in different parts of Tanzania, but their demography theses concentrate on the problem biologically and do not consider the psychological or sociological point of view.[38] There is only one study that focuses on the value of children and fertility. It concentrates on the economic value of children and deals only slightly with their non-economic value.[39]

Larsen and Raggers reveal in their study that infertility tends to be more prevalent in urban than in rural areas in sub-Saharan Africa. They maintain that this could result from the movement of infertile women away from their rural residences of origin to a more urban area.[40] The findings of Larsen and Raggers are interesting and sparked my desire to find out how it is in Kilimanjaro; whether there are any differences between the urban and rural situation for the life of infertile couples. I have not concentrated on finding out numbers of infertile couples in urban and rural Kilimanjaro; my main focus is to see if it is harder or easier to cope with infertility in a village community than in a town setting.

Many Western researchers concentrate on modern infertility cures in their studies. These studies are not central to the discourse of childlessness in Tanzania where these cures are generally not available. More useful to my study on Christian couples is the research that considers the psychosocial influence of infertility in the relationship between spouses.[41] The stress on psychosocial care of childless couples is a big issue in many Western countries. It is understood that the search for a medical cure is not enough. The crisis of infertility is a heavily psychological crisis where social support is often needed.

Most of the studies discussed above do not consider the personal experience of childlessness, but rather, concentrate on the phenomenon as such. Some more recent studies have considered the personal experience of childlessness. In many of these, the data consist of the life stories of infertile women. Marcia Inhorn's work focuses on poor urban Egyptians

---

38. Ngallaba, "Fertility Differentials"; Riwa, "Effect of Sex Preference"; Jiwani, "Use of Community-Level Data"; and Mtenga, "Value of Children."
39. Mtenga, "Value of Children."
40. Larsen and Raggers, "Levels and Trends," 46.
41. Miall, "Stigma"; Greil et al., "Infertility."

and analyzes infertility and patriarchy in family life in Egypt.[42] She focuses mainly on infertile women. Most of Inhorn's subjects are Muslims, but her study does give tools to interpret infertility in a Christian setting. She found her interviewees mainly through clinical settings and concentrated on the issue of medical cure. Even though the title of her book points to family life in Egypt, she mainly deals with the dilemma of childless wives. Inhorn's study was additionally useful while comparing the findings of the present study to the Egyptian situation.

Infertile Indian women have been studied by Catherine Kohler Riessman, who focuses on the narratives of individual women. The setting of hers studies is Kerala state in South India, the population of which is mainly Christian.[43] The personal experience of infertility and its effects on a marriage are interpreted well in Riessman's narratives, but she does not, however, deal much with the male perspective. Riessman and Inhorn found their subjects through various clinics and their interviews were mainly done in a clinical setting. Both Inhorn and Riessman had to rely on their research assistants' translations to such a degree that it sometimes raises questions about their interpretations.

The reproductive role of women in Tanzania is analyzed by Cuthbert K. Omari. He maintains that the status of a barren woman is low because the first priority of a wife is to bear children. Omari stresses that couples are not even able to make an independent decision over their own fertility because the influence of relatives is so strong.[44] He discusses the influence of barrenness on the status of women in a patriarchal society, and points to an important social aspect of the problem of infertility and family interference in Tanzania. His sociological strategy of dealing with the problem of infertility comes close to the approach of this study. He considers infertility a communal problem that affects the relationship of the couple and of the childless wife with her community. Omari does not, however, deal with male infertility.

Most of the studies on infertility concentrate on female infertility. There are few studies which have considered the male attitudes of fertility in various African countries.[45] All of these studies focused, however, mainly on men's desire for fertility, but they did not research male infertility as such.

42. Inhorn, *Infertility and Patriarchy*.
43. Riessman, "Personal Troubles."
44. Omari, "Fertility rates," 261.
45. Setel et. al, "Men's Perspectives"; Townsend, "Male Fertility"; Orobaton, "Dimensions of Sexuality."

Karina Kielmann has studied the identity of infertile women in a Muslim setting; in Pemba, in coastal Tanzania.[46] The culture of the coastal people in Pemba differs radically from that of the Chagga of Kilimanjaro. Kielmann did her field research in connection with a family health program in Pemba, and she herself criticizes the fact that the main interest of the health educators is to limit fertility and not to deal with those who have problems conceiving. Her study searched the context and consequences of female infertility. Kielmann's concentration on the concept of identity is valuable to the current study even though the setting differs considerably.

A discourse on infertility was studied by Zaida Mgalla and J. Ties Boerma, which was carried out in the Mwanza region of northwest Tanzania in the late 1990s.[47] The focus of their study is discussion among normal people about infertility. It reveals that cultural explanations such as witchcraft are more often supposed to be the reason for infertility than what the medical studies reveal. The insight for my study drawn from Mgalla and Boerma's research concerns this general interpretation of infertility. The Mwanza region, which is mainly populated by Sukumas, differs culturally from Kilimanjaro area, but people in Mwanza and Kilimanjaro area seem to share some aspects in their discourse on infertility. Another article on the same research project collected thirty life histories of women with infertility problems in Mwanza.[48] These life stories have been used only in a short article that does not narrate them in full detail. Both of these studies served as useful background material for my study of Christian couples in Kilimanjaro.

None of the above multidisciplinary studies on infertility focuses on Kilimanjaro. The first group, which focuses on population studies, guided me during the field research process. The second group, psychosocial studies of the life of infertile couples, contributed to the interpretation of findings. The third group, dealing with the life stories of infertile women, contributed especially to the style of writing, analysis, and the interpretation of narratives in this study. The fourth group, which consists of various studies on the impact of fertility and infertility on the life of women and men, contributed to my understanding of the communal nature of the problem of infertility in an African context. All these studies, however, avoided the pastoral side of the problem of infertility.

---

46. Kielmann, "Barren Ground."
47. Mgalla and Boerma, "Discourse of Infertility," 190.
48. Gijsels et. al., "'No Child Send.'"

Theological Research on Christian marriage in Africa

While population studies deal with the problem of childlessness in a secular context in society, theological research takes into account another important aspect of the community: the church. The church and its influence to the discussion regarding the value of children in Africa are further discussed below.

Many African theologians have dealt with the value of children in their writings. There are those who point to childlessness as the biggest curse in an African marriage and as a valid reason for either divorce or polygyny in a traditional society.[49] African theologians conclude that through marriage and procreation the African becomes immortal.[50] Marriage was and is understood as a process; an important part of this process is the birth of the first child. There are, however, other theologians who claim that African culture places too much emphasis on the role of children in a marriage.[51] According to these theologians, the harmful practices of African culture should not be followed in churches. Among the harmful practices which these female theologians include is the idea that the marriage is only for procreation. From their point of view, this understanding gives a woman only the role of reproduction, and leaves her without value as a human being.[52]

Various theological studies have given insight to the current study. The first group is Catholic theologians writing on Christian marriage in Africa, some specifically among the Chagga. The Catholic definition of marriage differs from the Lutheran, as was previously discussed in connection to Christian marriage in the Northern Diocese. For this reason, the Catholic contribution is less central to my study.

The second group of theologians studying Christian marriage is Lutheran Chagga theologians. Their contribution is more central to my own research because it deals with both the Chagga and the Lutheran contexts. These Lutheran studies, however, do not analyze the theology of marriage in a Chagga context very intensely.

The third group to be discussed in this section is the contribution of African feminist theologians concerning various marital problems. These feminist theologians discuss the practice of polygyny and other cultural practices which they consider to devalue women in Africa. Among

---

49. Mbiti, *African Religions*, 145.
50. Ibid., 110; Bahemuka, "Social Changes," 120.
51. Kanyoro, *Introducing Feminist Cultural Hermeneutics*, 69; Bahemuka, "Social Changes," 120–21.
52. Kanyoro, *Introducing Feminist Cultural Hermeneutics*, 69–70.

these feminist theologians, there is only one female theologian from the Northern Diocese and she is not of a Chagga origin. However, their contribution is important when studying the narratives of Christian couples from Machame. The fourth and last group is pastoral studies on infertility which are discussed at the end of this section. Their contribution is considerable, even though the data and scope of these studies differ from the current study.

Njuu, a Catholic Chagga theologian, deals with the cultural view of procreation and the Christian attitude towards the value of procreation. He comes to the conclusion that marriage is considered to be valid even when the couple is childless. Njuu searches the inculturation of the understanding of marriage in Kilimanjaro.[53] He is willing to unite the traditional values and the Christian teachings, but he does not give practical solutions as to how it would be possible.

Three other Catholic writers have contributed greatly to the discussion of Christian marriage in Africa. Benezeri Kisembo, Laurenti Magesa, and Aylward Shorter go further to discuss the consequences of infertility to a Christian marriage in Africa. They do not agree with those Roman Catholic writers who try to find a valid reason to dissolve a barren marriage. They continue to evaluate what the real meaning of a marriage is and they come to a conclusion that a childless union can be a sign of authentic married love.[54] Though not married themselves, these three Catholic priests know how hard it is to live in an African community without children. Kisembo et al. have important proposals for how the problem could be solved. What they lack is real empirical work on the life experiences of childless marriages.

Some Lutheran Chagga theologians deal with the value of children in Chagga society. They stress the importance of children, especially the need to have a male child, in the community. Jackson Malewo studied premarital counseling in the Northern Diocese. he deals mainly with the planning stage of Chagga marriage, and he touches on the problem of infertility in discussing premarital pregnancies. Malewo claims that the church teaches that marriage retains its value even in those cases where there are no children born into a family.[55] He does not, however, deal much with counseling for those already married. Malewo's contribution to my study is that he presents examples of marital problems in the Northern

---

53. Njuu,"Traditional Marriage," 21, 24.
54. Kisembo et. al., *African Christian Marriage,* 110–11.
55. Malewo, *Pre-marital Counseling,* 15–17.

Diocese. Among the major problems which Malewo refers to is the strong family interference.

Kaleb Shoo makes a comparison between the traditional Chagga marriage and Christian marriage in the Machame area.[56] Shoo's interesting ethnographic study of Machame traditions from the Nkwarungo area gave valuable background information to my study. Shoo maintains that the stability of the marriage depends on children. According to Shoo, children are regarded as a true link between the two families.[57]

A third Chagga pastor, Aaron Urio, deals with the concept of memory in the Chagga community. Urio maintains that barren persons are not remembered in the Chagga community after their death. In Urio's study, the importance of male children is stressed. Immortality in a patriarchal society is connected to the birth of a male child. Urio's approach is open for contextualization. When dealing with the concept of memory, Urio stresses the value of children to a Chagga marriage. He does not discuss the pastoral side of the problem of infertility. Urio emphasizes the importance of African immortality through procreation and touches on Christian immortality through Jesus Christ.[58] Urio's contribution to the current study is considerable. His theological and cultural analysis is profound and his interpretation of Chagga traditions and their influence on the life of the Lutheran church is valuable.

The Northern Diocese does not have a uniform theology of marriage. The three pastors of the Northern diocese discussed above have contributed to this discussion describing Chagga traditions and linking them directly to Christian practices. The Lutheran point of view remains unclear. Urio goes in the direction of contextual theology, but his topic is on Holy Communion as a memorial meal and so does not represent a contextual theology of marriage.

One female theologian of the Northern Diocese, Anastasia Malle, discusses the role of an African woman in marriage in her exegetical master's thesis on Hagar and in her dissertation on psalms of lament.[59] Malle concentrates in her field research on her own ethnic background, the Iraqw of the Karatu. Her findings shed light on the female interpretation of family situations in Tanzania.

---

56. Shoo, "Traditional African Marriage."
57. Ibid., 25.
58. Urio, *Concept of Memory*, 25.
59. Malle, "Hagar Names God"; "Interpreting the Lament Psalms."

Two feminist theologians from Kenya, Musimbi Kanyoro and Nyambura Njoroge, have dealt with marital practices in their writings.[60] Kanyoro and Njoroge stress that many marital practices harm the women of Africa and that these practices should not be followed in the Christian church. They are not against contextualization as such, but rather they want to stress that it is important to evaluate which African practices are good for the life of women in Africa and which practices harm and devalue women and girls. The findings of Kanyoro and Njoroge give important insight for the current study. Kanyoro's publication on *Feminist Cultural Hermeneutics*[61] is a valuable reference material in interpreting the narratives on childlessness in Machame. She acknowledges stories as an important tool for cultural hermeneutics in Africa. Her starting point is in Biblical stories, and she ends with interpretations of women's lives in western Kenya. My approach is to start from the life stories of Christian couples and to end with a more theoretical interpretation of the meanings of these narratives.

The need for counseling childless couples is raised by Nigerian Daisy Nwachuku. She argues that highly professionalized pastoral counseling sessions are needed to get down to the roots of the emotional burdens and problems of a childless couple within the Christian context.[62] Nwachuku points to an important need, even though her own study was conducted in a clinical setting. She notices the need to study childlessness in a Christian community and to counsel childless couples.

Shame is connected with childlessness, especially in Tanzanian communal cultures. Sylvester Kafunzile analyzed shame among the Haya women of northwestern Tanzania, and one of the sources that cause shame is barrenness. Kafunzile poses some important questions regarding family interference and its effect on childless couples in the Bukoba area, as well as on the role of barren women in Haya society.[63] Kafunzile's data is mainly from group interviews with Haya women, and he does not consider the male perspective on the shame of childlessness.

The above-mentioned theologians have dealt mainly with childlessness within African marriage. Childlessness has been frequently addressed but it has not been studied as a pastoral problem except in a few writings. The denominational background seems to make a difference in the ethical positions of these writers. The Roman Catholic theologians are more open to the

---

60. Kanyoro, *Introducing Feminist Cultural Hermeneutics*; Njoroge, "Groaning."
61. Kanyoro, *Introducing Feminist Cultural Hermeneutics*.
62. Nwachuku, "Rituals and Symbols," 82.
63. Kafunzile, "Shame," 104.

inculturation of the Christian marriage. The Lutheran theologians seem to be more hesitant to use the traditional values to justify their arguments.

The Aim of the Study

In the beginning of this study I concentrated on the role of a childless woman in her community. At that time I was interested in the influence of urbanization and social change on the attitudes towards childless women. As I continued with my field research, my main focus moved from studying the phenomenon of childlessness to concentrating on the personal experience of what it means for a person to live in the community without a child.

In the process of this study, the gender focus also changed. At first I presumed that childlessness affects mainly the life of women in Chagga society. Later I found it necessary to broaden my view and to concentrate on married couples in order to study how childlessness affects the marital life of contemporary Machame couples. Infertility has been seen as one of the main causes of marital breakdown in Africa in various studies.[64]

The aim of my research is to find out how a childless Christian couple constructs its identity in a Chagga community under the influence of three shifting cultural categories. This study researches the meaning of childlessness in the narrated life stories of childless couples and examines the coping strategies used. The focus is on the personal and communal narratives of the effects on childlessness in the marital life of Christian couples from Machame, in western Kilimanjaro. My main focus is neither on language nor on method as such. As a theologian, my interest is on the effects of childlessness to a marriage in a Christian community; thus by using narrative terms I will concentrate on the plot of these narratives. The purpose is to find out the role of the church in coping with the problem of infertility in the Chagga community. The role of pastors and other church workers is strong in the community, and my interest is to see how they influence the life of childless parishioners.

The aim discussed above indicates a gap in knowledge; childlessness in Christian community has not been studied as a theological and sociological problem. In addition to this, almost all recent studies have been conducted in eastern Kilimanjaro, which is culturally and linguistically different from the western side of the mountain; therefore, I have concentrated on western Kilimanjaro.

---

64. Mbiti, *Love and Marriage,* 197; Uka, "African Family," 195.

I

Research Procedure

The Field Research Communities

My goal was to find two parishes that were willing to accept my research proposal; one parish located close to Moshi town and a second that would be in a village area quite far from the influence of Moshi. I did not want to conduct my research in the center of the regional because many people come there from different parts of Kilimanjaro and some from outside the region altogether. Both of the chosen areas should preferably be on the same side of Moshi and to have cultural connections to each other.

I concentrated on the Machame cultural area in western Kilimanjaro. In the nineteenth and early twentieth century, the Machame area was a mission field of the German Leipzig Mission. The first missionaries who came to this area concentrated on the spiritual growth of the Christians.[1] They did not conduct wide anthropological studies, as their colleague Bruno Gutmann, of the same mission, did in the Old Moshi area. Gutmann was criticized by his fellow missionaries for being too bound to the social structures of the Chagga. The others, for example, the head of Leipzig Mission in Kilimanjaro, Johannes Raum, stressed the teaching and baptizing of the Chagga people.[2] The traditional practices, for example, female circumcision and ancestral sacrifices, seem to have been less common in the Machame area than in other parts of Kilimanjaro.[3] However, the traditional practices have influenced the life of the Chagga of Machame as well.

Two parishes in the eastern Hai District of the Northern Diocese, which is located on the southwestern slopes of Mount Kilimanjaro, were chosen to be the location of research. Both of these parishes belong to Nkwarungo, the main area of the old Machame kingdom and culture. The vernacular Kimachame and Machame traditions and background unite

---

1. Fleisch, *Lutheran Beginnings*, 48–50, 55–56; Smedjebacka, *Lutheran Church*, 36–38.
2. Shao, *Bruno Gutmann's Missionary Method*, 86.
3. Stambach, *Lessons*, 73–77, 153.

these two parishes. The difference between these parishes is that most of the parishioners in the rural parish were born in the area of the parish and truly belong to the Machame culture, whereas the area of the urban parish is more of a mixture of people from different places and backgrounds. These parishes will hereafter be referred to as the rural and the urban parish. For the sake of the anonymity of the interviewees, the parishes names and locations are withheld.

The population census of 1988 gives interesting figures on the population in northern and southern Machame. In southern Machame, where the urban parish is situated, the ratio of males to females is almost equal; there are only a few more men than women. In northern Machame, where the rural parish is, the male-female ratio is quite uneven, with a greater number of females than males.[4] This difference is attention grabbing given that the distance between these two parishes is barely ten kilometers. The main reason for the uneven number of males and females on the upper slopes of Kilimanjaro is that men have migrated to towns but most of the women have stayed in the villages.

The rural parish is located on the higher slopes of the mountain and consists of several villages. There are two churches in the parish and several other places of prayer. Most of the inhabitants in the area are Lutheran Christians, while only a couple of families are Muslims and a few others attend the Pentecostal churches on the lower slopes. The parishioners of the rural parish are mainly Chagga, born in Machame. Some people come from other parts of Tanzania; most of them are young paid workers on the Machame farms. Others who come from other ethnic backgrounds are married to Machame spouses. The main income of the parishioners comes from farming and cattle keeping. The higher slopes of Machame are famous for milk production. Parishioners in the rural parish are hardworking people who rest only on Sundays. During Sunday worship, the churches in the rural parish are full and the attendance consists of the old, middle-aged, and children. Most of the young people are either in schools or have migrated to towns in search of work. The scarcity of land does not offer employment to all the children in large families.

The urban parish is located on the lowland plain. The area is actually only semi-urban, into which most people have moved during the last twenty or thirty years. Before the 1960s, this area was a big field through which people traveled from the mountain to cultivate the land during the rainy seasons. Slowly, some members of the family moved permanently

---

4. See Tanzania National Bureau of Statistics, *Population Census* (1988), 51; "Hai District: Total Population" (2002).

into these villages closer to Moshi town. The urban parishioners consist of people of different occupations. Many are small-scale farmers, but in addition many are involved in various types of business, as the closeness of Moshi town increases the opportunities to do business.

Most people have moved to the urban parish from different parts of Machame, not only from Nkwarungo. Some people are from other parts of Kilimanjaro and from other ethnic groups. The Lutherans in this area are mostly from Machame, while the Roman Catholic population is mostly from the Kibosho area, the neighboring kingdom of Machame towards the east. In the Kilimanjaro area, the connection between ethnic and language identity and religious denomination membership can be clearly seen. Ethnic identity is not a clear denominational division in that all Chaggas are Lutherans or even Christians, but most people from Kilema, Kibosho, and Rombo are Roman Catholics and most people from Machame, Marangu, and Mwika are Lutherans. Language identity in different parts of Kilimanjaro is different; the various Chagga dialects are almost different languages. Kimachame is closer to Kimeru, a vernacular that is spoken among the Meru people, than it is to the Kichagga of Mwika of eastern Kilimanjaro.

In the area of the urban parish there are also some Chaggas who are Muslims, many of whom come from Machame area. There are also Pentecostal churches in this area, most of the adherents being converts from the Lutheran and the Roman Catholic churches. When I compare the religious pluralism that exists in the urban parish to the almost monolithic Lutheranism in the rural parish, the religious situation is very different. The religious difference can also be seen inside the Lutheran church, as when observing the confirmation celebrations in both of the studied parishes. The confirmation is celebrated in a much more simple way in the rural parish; it does not allow girls to dress up like brides in a wedding. The confirmation in the urban parish looks, from a distance, like a wedding of many small brides.

After the decision was made to concentrate on these two parishes, I used my personal contacts to be introduced to their workers and lay leaders. One pastor, a friend of mine who works in the Northern Diocese, introduced me to the leading pastor of the urban parish. He took my research request to the parish council and I was given permission to conduct interviews among the parishioners. One of my students was doing her internship in the rural parish, where, when I visited her there, I was introduced for the first time. I asked for research permission from them and after few months I was given permission to conduct interviews.

Collection of the Data

Participant Observation and Preparatory Interviews

I used triangulation of various qualitative data collection methods in order to collect a variety of valid data.[5] Participant observation had three phases during the field research process, and different types of interviews followed one another as new needs and strategies arose.

Participant observation involves social interaction between the researcher and informants. The aim of participant observation is to collect systematic data on the life situation of informants.[6] I agree with Kvale who claims that such observation will give more valid knowledge of people's behavior and their interaction with their environment than with other data collection methods.[7] Another important quality of participant observation is that it is an open-ended and flexible process of inquiry.[8]

Pre-fieldwork participant observation was done mainly in the field before selecting people to be interviewed.[9] I used this period of observation as orientation to the field. I offered my help to preach in worship services and was, in this way, introduced to all parishioners. Preaching was an efficient strategy to establish rapport with the informants. Many of the interviewees remembered me from the church service when I approached them later. They knew me and clearly trusted me, even though I did not always recognize them from among the thousand or so parishioners who gathered for a full confirmation service.

I used focused observation during the early period of field research.[10] During the second phase of observation, I observed people's lives in worship services, during ceremonies such as weddings, send-offs, and confirmations, as well as in their homes. Visits to women's groups and observations during other activities at the church helped me to meet as many people in both communities as possible. Frequently I tried to visit the church workers to get to know them better and to gain more information about the parishes. After I had met people a few times, it was easier to select interviewees and to conduct interviews in a good atmosphere. During this period I only did some group interviews and had many informal discussions. The main research interviews were done only after the

---

5. Flick, *Introduction*, 226.
6. Taylor and Bogdan, *Introduction*, 15.
7. Kvale, *Interviews*, 98, 104.
8. Flick, *Introduction*, 139–40.
9. Taylor and Bogdan, *Introduction*, 16–75; Flick, *Introduction*, 140.
10. Flick, *Introduction*, 140.

contacts had been established with the community and after the people got to know me.

When observing and participating in the life of the studied communities I had opportunity to establish rapport with my informants, however, this rapport did not come quickly. It took time before people would open up to me and accept my visits. When creating rapport I used many different strategies.[11] One important topic of common interest that I discussed was animal husbandry and farming. The Chagga are very hardworking people and proud of their work on the farms. I enjoyed learning a lot during the times I spent on their farms or when observing groups of women drying their garden products in the sun.

During the third phase of observation, I chose to observe the childless couples and their lives. My aim was to find further evidence of the influence of childlessness on their lives. Many of the childless couples whom I met did not have anything against informal discussions and my observations. I observed that men had more difficulty in sharing their feelings about childlessness.

I finished each phase of observation when I felt it could not provide any further insights or knowledge.[12] During the observation, opportunities for interviews arose spontaneously from the regular field contacts[13] and the preparatory interviews were done during the first two phases of observation.

Before entering the field, I made some pilot interviews outside the studied communities to gain experience on the topic, on terminology, and on the way of conducting interviews in an African setting. The pilot interviews were conducted with my students of the spouses class at Makumira University College. After these few pilot interviews, I had an idea of people's reactions to my questions and found out which questions were too structured and prevented me from getting people's own ideas.

Some experts outside the two parishes were also interviewed before the actual research interviews took place so as to gain wider knowledge of family issues and Chagga traditions. I interviewed various experts in order to gain background information to help plan the right interview questions. Among these experts was the leader of women's desk in Northern Diocese and a lawyer who works for KWIECO (Kilimanjaro Women Information and Exchange Consultancy), a nongovernmental organization supporting women in Kilimanjaro region. I also had informal discussions with

---

11. Taylor and Bogdan, *Introduction*, 36–38.
12. Flick, *Introduction*, 136.
13. Ibid., 90.

medical personnel from the head office of the Northern Diocese and from Machame Hospital. I visited the KIWAKKUKI (Kikundi cha Wanawake wa Kilimanjaro Kupambana na Ukimwi) women's group, which works for AIDS-affected people in Kilimanjaro region, and NAFGEM (Network Against Female Genital Mutilation). Some of these background interviews contributed significantly to the planning of actual research questions; others were nice visits to various places without producing much useful input for my study.

The first interviews in the field were group interviews with the women's group that meets once a week in both study parishes.[14] During three occasions in late 1999 and early 2000, I met more than fifty women and had a chance to fix a date for further interviews with a few of them. These group discussions were a great opportunity to gain more information on the Machame traditions and the general attitudes of women toward marital issues. There was no possibility of having a very personal and deep discussion because of the presence of so many people. The group interview data was used as additional information to interpret the personal interview data collected during the latter two phases of personal interviews.

Observations and group discussions were a two-way learning and sharing experience. I learned from the parishioners and their lifestyle, but they also wanted to learn from me regarding family matters in Finland. During the group discussions I faced, for example, questions on marital practices, the attitude of the Lutheran church in Finland toward divorce, and on official adoption and how it is organized in my country. An important part of this time was the sharing of experiences of motherhood with these Chagga mothers. Women in the parishes were interested in hearing about my children and the way I raise them.

Observations and those interviews that were not tape-recorded are documented in three fieldwork diaries. The first diary covers the period from December 1999 until January 2001. The second diary covers February and March 2002. I kept the two small diaries in my bag and wrote notes in them mainly after I had left a place. I completed the notes as soon as I left the venue of observation, and later, during the same evening or at latest the following morning, I completed full diary notes. I also recorded my own remarks and things that I did not understand in these full diary notes.[15] The third diary, which is bigger in size, contains notes from November 2001 until February 2002. I used this seminar notebook

---

14. Ibid., 127–28.
15. Ibid., 168.

for those occasions where writing notes was natural, such as in seminars or during formal interviews.

The notes from all three fieldwork diaries helped me to continue with my interviews, and the recorded remarks have been very valuable information when analyzing my data. Informal conversations on childlessness went on during the whole process of research with many men, women, and youngsters. Many of these informal conversations are also documented in the fieldwork diaries.

Two Phases of Personal Interviews

In the beginning of the first phase of personal interviews, many people recommended that I should interview the old people in the community who knew the history and traditions of the Chagga of Machame. Some of these interviews with elders were interesting, but from others I only gained background information on different traditions and not much on the topic of study. Many of the Chagga elders were not ready to reveal the problems in their communities to an outsider but wanted to talk only about the good things in their culture. Culturally, it is not acceptable to discuss problems in the community with an outsider, and the elders were behaving correctly according to this precept.

The first phase of personal interviews consisted of ethnographic interviews with parishioners and church workers.[16] I conducted the interviews during the 2000–2001 academic year. The initial topic of these interviews regarded the value of children. After speaking about the value of children, I asked more on the situation of not having children in a Lutheran Chagga marriage. After discussing that, I focused on questions regarding infertility treatments, counseling, influence of infertility on a marriage and on relationships in the family and larger community, funeral practices of childless members of the communities, and identities and status of childless individuals in the interviewee's community. The total number of interviews during the first phase was thirty-three; among them were the four first person interviews.

My role was quite active during the ethnographic, thematic interviews. Most of the interviews of the first phase were dialogical and consisted of many question-answer transitions. The content of these interviews followed a thematic pattern, where the starting point was the discussion about the value of children in Machame. The length of these ethnographic interviews varied from fifteen minutes to two hours. The data from these

---

16. Ibid., 127–28.

interviews contributed background information to the narratives of this study; some of them contained complete narratives on the life of childless couples in Machame.

After the first phase I was not satisfied with the content of interviews. The discussions reached a far too abstract level, and only when people referred directly to their own or somebody else's life experiences did the interviews reveal the influence of childlessness within marriage. There was a need for new interview strategy. I founded the narrative approach, further discussed in the section below entitled "Narrative Analysis Rises from the Oral Tradition," after hesitating with the results of the first phase.

The second phase of interviews took place during the 2001–2002 academic year. Many of these life story interviews were first person narratives of a childless life. I continued, however, to conduct third person interviews in order to gain knowledge on the reaction of the community towards childless marriages. From this point on, I divide the narratives collected during the personal interviews into first- and third-person narratives. The total number of life story interviews was eleven, among them six personal life stories of childless persons and three personal life stories of single mothers. Three people were interviewed during both of the phases, among them one first-person and two third-person narrators.

My role was more that of an active listener in the life story interviews. I followed the advice of Robert Atkinson on how to conduct narrative interviews that concentrate on life stories. Atkinson stresses the use of an open-ended interview approach in the life story interviews, where specific questions are asked only when help is needed to guide the narrator to continue her or his narrative.[17] I did not have a prepared structure for my interviewees; I conducted all the interviews myself and did not feel the need to have a clear structure.

I wanted to create a good atmosphere in which the interviewee had a freedom to narrate. Atkinson gives advice on how to create a good narrative; using photographs, for example, to help people to recall the stories and events in their lives.[18] In some cases I looked at photographs with an interviewee, in other cases that did not seem appropriate to the situation. The open strategy resulted, in an African setting, to invite interviewees to provide rich life stories. Many of the life story interviews were quite monological and provided almost a complete narrative.[19] Other narrators, especially men and some women who were not especially talented narra-

---

17. Atkinson, *Life Story Interview*, 31.
18. Ibid., 31.
19. Lieblich et al., *Narrative Research*, 26.

tors, provided a sparse narrative of their life. Such narratives were often, however, compact and informative even though short.

During the life story interviews, my strategy was even more unstructured. My way of conducting interviews was very informal; they were more of a sharing of experiences with different people than sterile research interviews. I found out that this more informal approach made people relax and talk more freely. I used broad questions in order to give the individual freedom to reply, making the situation more like a conversation.[20] When people relaxed, I became more active in listening and less active in talking. I encouraged the interviewees to continue their story by nonverbal or paralinguistic expressions of interest and attention such as a slight nod or "mhm." I mainly used one starting question: "Would you tell me about your life?" Or, in the cases of third person interviews, I could ask, "Would you tell me about a life of a certain childless couple in the community?" During the life story interviews, I raised some further questions when needed. I wanted to hear of marital life, of the life of a childless person in the African family and in the larger community, of funeral plans and the understanding of immortality, and of questions such as regarding adoption and fosterage. Some of the life story interviews were short and concise, but most of them were long and included many small stories. These stories were not told in a chronological order and, in order to understand the life stories, I had to ask some clarifying questions about times and places. I conducted the interviews on my own with the interviewee/s.

Conducting interviews in Tanzania was very time-consuming work. Many times I had to make two or three trips just to interview one person. During the first trip I fixed a time with an interviewee or asked somebody else to make sure that the person knew when I would be coming to interview her/him. When I made the second trip to conduct the interview, many times the person could not come at all or was late to arrive at the agreed interview place. Because of this I could not plan to have many interviews on a single day, usually only one or two.

The agricultural cycle influenced the timing of interviews. I conducted most of my interviews in January and February, after the busy Christmas season but before the planting season of big rains in March–April. Another good time to conduct interviews was October–November, which is after harvesting but before Christmas.

In Machame it is not polite to visit people without having somebody to escort and introduce you. In some cases, a gatekeeper escorted me to meet a certain person. In the beginning of field research, church

---

20. Riessman, *Narrative Analysis*, 55.

workers took the role of a gatekeeper to introduce me to the parishioners. Later in the research process when I already knew many people, I asked the previous interviewees to help to introduce me to new people. This research strategy is called "snow-balling," and can be effectively used to obtain access to private settings. The aim is to start with a small number of people and win their trust, then to ask them to introduce you to others. It was more informal to go to a home with a neighbor to escort me than with a pastor of the parish. Taylor and Bogdan consider what a researcher should say to gatekeepers about the study and advise not to reveal details concerning the research.[21] I told the leading pastors of both parishes that I was interested to learn about the life of childless couples, while other gate keepers were only told that I do research in family issues.

Interruptions happened often when interviewing in homes, but this is part of normal life in Tanzania and it did not affect the situation very much. Members of the family, and many times neighbors, came to greet and to pass by during interviews, but they did not usually interrupt the secrecy of the sensitive issues discussed. During these interruptions I turned off the tape recorder and the interview continued after visitors left the room.

Many of the interviews were conducted in an empty meeting room at a church, which was seen as a neutral and quiet place. This is especially true for women for whom it is hard to meet in homes where they are always busy and unable to concentrate on talking for a long time with a visitor. When the meeting took place at the church, female interviewees could concentrate better than when in their own home.

The long field research process increased the validity of the data. It helped me to build rapport with the parishioners in Machame and enabled me to observe the marital life in the studied communities. The thorough field research process also enabled me to find new, more efficient ways of collecting data.

Basic Features of the Sample

The data used in this study comes from oral, personal interviews on childlessness in Machame. The notes from participant observation and from group interviews are used only as background information to interpret the data from personal interviews. The total number of personal interviews is forty-two. Most of them are tape-recorded (thirty-eight); only four are documented using only notes, but one of these, an interview of a childless

---

21. See Taylor and Bogdan, *Introduction*, 24–25.

spouse, was later reinterviewed using a tape recorder. For the validity of interpretation, the high acceptance of recording was important.

The data of this study is not a statistically balanced sample, as there are too few subjects and they were not chosen randomly, but specifically. Since the focus is on narratives of childless couples in Machame, the interviewees had to be chosen selectively. Three groups of people were selected for interviews in order to get the full picture of childlessness as a pastoral problem. The childless couples were selected because they were known to be childless. Normal parishioners and the workers of these parishes were selected because they could explain the attitudes towards childlessness and give third-person narratives on the experience of these childless individuals.

The first group of interviewees consists of married men and women parishioners who are, or were previously, unable to have children. In two cases, I interviewed both the husband and the wife/wives. In the first case a husband and his former wife were interviewed separately. In the second case were all of the spouses present during an interview, this being when I interviewed a polygynist man and his two wives. Among other couples I interviewed only one of the spouses. Women were more willing to accept my interview request, and also had more time to be interviewed.

The second group is that of ordinary parishioners of both sexes and all ages except children and youth. I decided not to include children and youth in this study after meeting with some of them in their schools and during confirmation lessons. Informal discussion with them revealed that they young people were not ready to be interviewed on family matters. Those in this group included friends, neighbors, colleagues, and relatives of the childless persons interviewed. They have a variety of occupational and educational backgrounds; among them are teachers, small-scale farmers, businessmen, nurses, a carpenter, and a builder. Many are church elders or are otherwise active in church activities, for example, in choirs. Others have been less active parishioners.

The last group I interviewed consists of church workers, including pastors, evangelists, parish workers, and kindergarten teachers. I interviewed six who were, at the time of the research, working in the urban parish. Additionally, I interviewed two people who had earlier worked in the parish; one of these used to work in the urban parish but has now retired, and the other now serves in a different parish in the Northern Diocese. In the rural parish I interviewed three church workers who are presently employed by the parish, and two others who had earlier worked in the same parish but are currently posted in other parishes of the Northern Diocese.

Many of these workers are, at the same time, personal friends or neighbors of the childless couples in the community, and some of them are relatives. The table below shows how the interviews were distributed among the interview groups, men and women, and the two study parishes.

Table 1: Interviewees in two study parishes

Parish	CP F	CP M	CP Total	P F	P M	P Total	CW F	CW M	CW Total	Total
Rural	3	2	5	4	3	7	1	4	5	17
Urban	2	-	2	12	1	13	3	5	8	23
Total	5	2	7	16	4	20	4	9	13	40

CP = Childless person   P = Parishioner   CW = Church worker

There were both men and women interviewed in each of the three groups. The ratio of males is largest in the group of church workers, which is fitting because most pastors and evangelists are men. The majority of those in the parishioner and childless person groups are women.

The age of the interviewees was considered in the selection criteria. The youngest person was in her twenties and the oldest was over ninety years of age. In Table 2 I have divided the interviewees into those younger than forty-five and those forty-five and older. In Chagga culture, forty is considered to be still on the younger side of adulthood, and many this age still have young children. Forty-five, however, is about the age at which some Chagga become grandparents, and also about the age at which childbearing becomes very rare.

Table 2: Distribution of Age

Group	Under 45	45 and over	Total
Childless	1	6	7
Parishioners	2	18	20
Church workers	6	7	13
Total	9	31	40

Most of the interviewees were born in the Machame area. Some were born in other parts of Kilimanjaro, and only one was born outside of Kilimanjaro, in the neighboring Meru area. Most of those coming from other parts of Kilimanjaro are women who married men from Machame. These wives have an understanding of the Machame culture through their husbands and in-laws, and many of them have learned the vernacular *kimachame*. Since they themselves were born in other parts of Kilimanjaro, many of them can analyze the differences between the traditions in Machame and in their original home place. All other interviewees belong to the Chagga ethnic group, except for one Meru woman who is married to a man from Machame. In summary, all of the interviewees are members of the studied communities, whether through birth or through marriage or work in Machame, and they have become full members of the parishes and neighborhoods in which they live.

Table 3: Place of Birth

Group	Machame	Kilimanjaro	Meru	Total
Childless individuals	4	3		7
Parishioners	12	7	1	20
Church workers	9	4		13
Total	25	14	1	40

Because the chosen communities are Lutheran parishes, all except one of the interviewees are Lutherans. This one exception is a childless person who is Roman Catholic but lives in the area of the urban parish and in the Lutheran neighborhood. I wanted to concentrate on Lutheran Christians because Catholics and Muslims have different understandings of marriage. For this reason Catholics and Muslims are not considered full members of the Lutheran communities studied even though they live within the area.

My Role as a Researcher

I wanted to find balance between having some commitment in the field communities and retaining a scientific distance.[22] I have used the "etic" position, where I, as an outsider, analyze narratives in the studied communities using outside concepts and phenomena. "Emic" typology, where one looks at people and their attitudes completely from inside, would not have been possible because the people themselves do not often see how deeply their traditional culture and religion continues to influence their behavior.[23]

---

22. Flick, *Introduction*, 54.
23. Pike, *Language in Relation*, 53.

I solved the dilemma of participation by taking the role of a "marginal insider."[24] Because of my status and work as a pastor, I was invited to join these communities as a regular visitor. This level of participation in the Lutheran community qualified me as a marginal insider. To be a full member of these local communities requires one to have been born in the Machame area or to marry somebody from there.

As a European, I will always be an outsider to some degree in an African context, but not necessarily a stranger.[25] However, it should be noted that my status of being a foreigner frequently helped me during my research. People were more open to talk to me about their personal experiences because of that distinction. They knew they would not have to face me every day and remember the things they had told me. They also understood that I could ask funny questions because I did not know the culture of the people very well.

I also used my role as a foreigner as a strategy to request recording. Interviewees accepted the request of tape recording when I explained that I needed to use it in order to have the possibility of checking the contents afterwards with a dictionary.

My identity as a pastor was both advantageous and, at times, problematic. It incorporated me quickly into the communities as a marginal insider and yet it identified me with the church only. In the beginning of my research this was a great advantage, but later it became an occasional burden, especially when I wanted to discuss traditional practices. The Lutheran church in the Machame area openly teaches that the traditional practices are against Christian teachings. As a result of this, if Christians practice traditional beliefs they have to do it secretly. Consequently, many were not easily willing to discuss their traditional beliefs with a visiting pastor who they feared might share their story with the church.[26]

As a woman I had natural and effective contacts with women of different ages. My role as a wife and a mother of three children has helped me in talking about marital questions with people. Even though I was considered to be young, people treated me as an adult because of my status as a mother. Also, those interviewees who do not have children themselves have found it natural that I have children myself.

My contact with men was also quite easy. As a pastor, my role was quite neutral in these communities. In the Northern Diocese there are many female pastors, and they are respected and well accepted in the community.

24. See Freilich, "Toward a Formalization," 536–39.
25. Stambach, *Lessons*, 47.
26. Ibid., 73.

Among the Chagga, the gender roles are quite fixed, but pastors, especially white women, are generally treated more like men. People are used to the male-like behavior of white women and accept their more active role. Many times, for example, when eating together, I ate with the men indoors while the other women ate outdoors, as the tradition dictates.

My experience with clinical pastoral counseling in four different Finnish hospitals helped me in conducting interviews on such a sensitive issue as childlessness. The context may have been different, but often the situation was quite similar as when I did clinical pastoral counseling in 1992. Like patients in Finnish hospitals, interviewees in Kilimanjaro needed a person whom they felt could they could trust and who listened attentively. Many interviewees were a bit nervous in the beginning and commented to me, "Ask the next question, ask!" Likewise, many patients in Finland were nervous when a pastor came to visit them in the hospital. Some of them exclaimed, "I am not dying yet!" Some of the childless interviewees had a similar reaction when they saw me for the first time: "Who has told you that I have a problem? Go away and do not bother me!" After discussing and sharing my own personal experiences of having to wait for my first child, many of them finally agreed to be interviewed.

The sharing of personal information was often a two-way street. I visited people in their homes and during their activities at church. Some parishioners and church workers visited us in Makumira. My experience of many years in Tanzania certainly helped my role as a researcher. Knowing, at least most of the time, when to speak and when to keep quiet helped me build confident relationships with the people in the studied communities.

Narrative Analysis Rises from the Oral Tradition

Chagga Oral Tradition Directs Towards Using Narrative Analysis

In the Chagga society, as in many other African societies, oral tradition is an important instrument in adaptive learning. This oral tradition contains many different forms: riddles, proverbs, songs, folktales, historical narratives, and myths.[27] In Chagga society, riddles that challenge the listener to explore experience in order to discover further meaning are widely used in normal conversation, even today. Many of the historical narratives and myths that are not commonly remembered were fortunately collected in the written Chagga ethnographies.[28]

---

27. Shorter, *African Culture*, 57–59.
28. Stahl, *History of the Chagga*.

Even though part of the oral tradition is no longer well known, the background of this tradition has influenced people's way of communicating. The Chagga grow up hearing tales and riddles, and the younger generation still uses stories as a way of communication. The Chagga more freely talk about sensitive issues when using narratives. Traditionally, the way of talking about rites of initiation or fertility among the Chagga has been through proverbs or riddles.[29] Also of note, the value of humor in the narrative tradition is very important. When using humor in sensitive issues, the narrative does not appear to be too serious.[30]

Sambuli Mosha, a Chagga scholar, describes the formative role of narration. He defines the meaning of a story for the Chagga as the potential to teach both oneself and others. Mosha analyzes in his study the use of narratives in Chagga history but claims that the oral tradition continues to be an important part of informal education. He further claims that storytelling is one of the most powerful and effective means for a holistic education in indigenous Chaggaland.[31] Mosha stresses the importance of narratives in education, but also notes that narratives are used for other purposes.

Traditionally, Chagga tales and myths were shared with large audiences during evening fires. The time chosen for stories is important: evening is the best time because work has stopped and it is the time to relax.[32] People enjoy telling stories to a large audience, and when they do their stories tend to be filled with more humor and horror than when they are told to just one person.[33] I saw the effect of the presence of a group in the beginning of my field research when I discussed family traditions with women's groups in the parishes. In these group discussions, some of the women emerged as artists of oral tradition while others gathered to make an audience for their stories.

Life stories, especially concerning the difficult parts of life, are not stories to be shared in groups. Stories of childlessness are family secrets and, therefore, are told either as gossip (which I did not prefer) or as personal or family narratives to be spoken of in a quieter setting. During the group interviews some interviewees gossiped about childless couples, but other participants corrected them and told them not to exaggerate.

29. Raum, *Chaga Childhood*.
30. Okpewho, *Epic in Africa*, 2, 202–39.
31. Mosha, *Heartbeat*, 48–49.
32. Ibid., 51.
33. Okpewho, *Epic in Africa*, 2, 240; Finnegan, *Oral Literature*, 2–6.

Narrative analysis suits the Tanzanian situation extremely well because of the prevalence of oral tradition. People enjoy telling stories, both their own life stories and those of others. It is easier to analyze the deeper meaning through their stories than from their replies to interview questions.

When I began my first phase of personal interviews, I did not have any idea about narrative analysis. When I was conducting my interviews I noticed that people replied to my open questions by using stories. People also wanted to teach me about their culture through telling me stories, and they used riddles in order to check if I had understood the deeper meaning. With their stories in mind, I started to search for a suitable method of collecting and analyzing the data.

My research needed a methodology that would not merely seek facts and events, but would reveal the ways such narrated events suggested an individual's relationship to the society in which she/he lives. Narrativity as an analytic perspective gives voice to the small people. Therefore, for my study narrative analysis worked well in giving a voice to the childless, who do not dare to speak about their problems in their own communities.

What Is Narrative Analysis?

Narrative research refers to any study that uses or analyses narrative data.[34] I understand narrative analysis both as a method for conducting interviews, which was previously explained in connection to life story interviews, and also as a method for analyzing the gathered material. Thus, narrative analysis has to do with how texts are interpreted; however, there is more than one method of doing narrative analysis. In order to understand this variety, let us first examine the history of narrative analysis.

There is a long history in the humanities of studying stories and autobiographies. Already in the 1960s many scholars of literature studies addressed narrative. Many of those who studied semiotics concentrated on narratives, and by the end of 1960s linguists had formulated a theory of how to analyze personal stories. There was research and discussion about narrative in these and other disciplines, but it was done separately, without interdisciplinary cooperation.[35]

The big change came in the 1980s, often considered the period of the "narrative turn," when various disciplines became interested in narrative analysis.[36] During that decade there were three important publications that invented what we today call "narrative analysis." In 1981, for the

---

34. Lieblich et al., *Narrative Research*, 2.
35. Lieblich et al., *Narrative Research*, 3–6; Riessman, *Narrative Analysis*, 1.
36. Riessman, *Narrative Analysis*, 1.

first time, there was an interdisciplinary effort to unite the different fields that had undertaken the study of narratives. W. T. Mitchell edited a book which included articles from Victor Turner and Paul Ricoeur, among others. [37] Also in 1981, Alasdair McIntyre emphasized that human identity is built and exists in the form of narrative.[38] McIntyre drew out the fact that people live out their narratives—it is not only a matter of telling stories. The third important publication in the history of narrative analysis is Paul Ricoeur's large project *Time and Narrative*. Ricoeur's main aim was to unite the philosophical and historical interpretation of narratives. All three of these studies made a difference to earlier narrative studies. Suddenly it was not only a question of studying them but living them, and, as a result, creating new stories.

Since the early 1980s there has been a narrative boom. Scholars of various fields have expressed their interest in narratives and have started to use narrative analysis as a way of doing research. Today we understand narrative analysis not as a single binding theory but as a loose group of methods and theories with great conceptual diversity that concentrate on the study of narrative. There are various ways of doing narrative analysis, and each researcher formulates his/her way of applying it.[39] The influence of postmodernism in the humanities and, later, in the social sciences is clearly seen in today's concentration on narrative. Kvale claims that there is openness to qualitative diversity and to the multiplicity of meanings in local contexts. Collective stories contribute to upholding the values of the community.[40]

Lieblich et al. have grouped three major ways of using narrative analysis: in the investigation of any research question, in studies that investigate narrative as their research object, and studies on the philosophy and methodology of narrative research. The first group includes those studies where narrative is used to represent the lifestyle of a specific group in a society. The second group consists of studies in literature and linguistics, where the main focus is on the form of narrative. The third group includes various books on methods of conducting narrative research.[41]

---

37. Mitchell, *On Narrative*.
38. McIntyre, *After Virtue*.
39. Riessman, *Narrative Analysis*, 5, 17.
40. Kvale, *Interviews*, 42–43.
41. Lieblich et al., *Narrative Research*, 3–6.

Locating Myself in Narrative Theory

Theologians, especially biblical scholars, were among the first to concentrate on narrative. According to Dan A. Stiver, there are three main schools of narrative theologians in the U.S., where narrative theology first emerged.[42] The first on his list is the California school, which is distinguished by its emphasis on correlation between the Christian's life story and the biblical narrative. As a result, pastoral issues and spirituality occupy a central role in this theological thinking.[43] One important contributor in the California school is James McClendon. He describes the task of theology as the study of how individuals and communities live their Christian faith.[44]

The second school, according to Stiver, is comprised researchers at Yale, notably Hans W. Frei, who claims that the purpose of biblical narratives is to define the identity of the subject, the reader him/herself.[45] The starting point for the Yale school is the biblical narratives themselves. Another whose contribution in the Yale school is central is George W. Lindbeck, who argues that believers make the story of the Bible their story. It is the text which absorbs the world, rather than vice versa.[46] The school of Yale makes a clear distinction between the disciplines of theology and philosophy.

For the third school of narrative theologians, the Chicago school, the starting point is narrativity itself, which is later used in order to interpret the Bible. Paul Ricoeur, noted previously, is the most famous among the Chicago school, which differs from the Yale school in claiming that it is impossible to come to a final or authoritative interpretation of a text. According to the Chicago school, interpretation is like a spiral in which we start with understanding and move interpretation, and then return again to understanding.[47] The Chicago school does not concentrate only on biblical interpretation but claims that narrativity opens up the possibility to understand and to interpret various narratives. Most narrative theologians belonging to the Chicago school are systematic theologians who do not separate themselves from other disciplines but are open, for example, to philosophical analysis.

---

42. Stiver, *Philosophy of Religious Language*, 134–62.
43. Navone, *Seeking God in Story*, 289–90.
44. McClendon, *Biography as Theology*.
45. Frei, *Eclipse of Biblical Narrative*, 135, 311, 323–24.
46. Lindbeck, *Nature of Doctrine*, 118.
47. Stiver, *Philosophy of Religious Language*, 101–3, 135.

The present study has been influenced mostly by the California school because it shares my interest in pastoral issues while concentrating on life stories. The school of Chicago has, however, given tools to interpret the personal experiences of my subjects in Kilimanjaro through its open attitude towards various disciplines. My approach differs from the Yale school in that I concentrate on life stories and do not use the biblical story as the starting point. Another major difference is that the present study does not concentrate on linguistic analysis, the main focus of the Yale school.

There is considerable disagreement about the definition and use of the basic terms in narrative research. According to Donald Polkinghorne, the term *narrative* refers specifically to texts that are thematically organized by plots.[48] Polkinghorne's definition does not reveal the difference between a narrative and a story, both of which are organized by plots. A useful distinction for my present study was Alexandra Georgakopoulou's analysis of small stories. She points out that a small story is a part of a bigger narrative. In her point of view, small stories often tend to be ignored. That is because they contain everyday information which the researchers consider trivial and not contributing to identity formation. Georgakopoulou argues that these small stories actually contribute significantly to a person's identity construction.[49]

I use the term *narrative* to point to those model narratives that are constructed from the small stories told by interviewees in Kilimanjaro. Thus, the term narrative points to model narratives of the final report; a *story* refers to an authentic part of a life story from an interview in those cases where there is a plot. I call those authentic descriptions that are not plotted *accounts* or *explanations*. Riessman claims that not all narratives in interviews are plotted.[50] My interviewees expressed themselves using accounts communicated with or without plot; both contained important meanings and interpretations of the marital life of childless couples.

In this study, narrative analysis functions as a method for analyzing stories in order to produces paradigmatic typologies or categories.[51] Through these typologies, in my case the model stories, analysis is presented to the reader first in the form of model narratives and later in theoretical viewpoints that reveal the meaning of these model narratives. The life stories are both the starting point and the final result of the study in narrative analysis. This is one of the biggest differences from the previous

---

48. Polkinghorne, "Narrative Configuration," 5.
49. Georgakopoulou, "Thinking Big with Small Stories," 123.
50. Riessman, *Narrative Analysis*, 18.
51. Polkinghorne, "Narrative Configuration," 5–6.

methods of studying stories and autobiographies, as traditional methods did not see the importance of producing new stories as a result of study.

There are, however, many narrative scholars who disagree with the use of anything other than authentic first-person accounts as data for narrative research.[52] There are also those who do use narratives to represent a larger group. Sintonen, for example, interviewed many Finnish immigrant men in Canada, but in his research report he chose to present only two life narratives, Eino I and Eino II. [53] Sintonen's presentation differs from mine in that the two life stories he uses are authentic stories, not constructed narratives like the model narratives of this study. He also uses only first-person accounts, whereas I also use third-person accounts of life stories. Sintonen's decision to use only two of the stories to represent the other stories at large shows, however, that he does not follow the strong postmodern trend of many narrative scholars who emphasize that an experience is always spontaneous and personal.

Another topic that divides narrative scholars is the question of narrative representation of experience. I join those narrative scholars who believe that narratives provide us with access to the interviewee's identity.[54] Some narrative scholars are of that opinion that the identity presented in a narrative actually is the narrator's personal identity.[55] Considering my data, I would think that this is too strong a claim to make. My starting point was the personal and communal narratives of childless couples, and the result was an interpretation of identity in Machame. In my view, the narratives of the childlessness in Machame reveal something about identity and its systems of meaning in that culture.[56] These narrative identities are not, however, people's complete personal or communal identities in Machame. Personal life narratives change during the course of life. The life narratives of this research are only like static pictures and not like a video which is moving.[57]

There are a huge number of narrative studies that concentrate on identity in one way or other. The difference between the two sides of personal identity is evaluated by Paul Ricoeur. On one side, identity is sameness, while on the other side, identity is selfhood. Sameness concerns how the individual is related to the community. Selfhood refers to the way a person

---

52. Riessman, *Narrative Analysis*, 1.
53. Sintonen, *Etninen identiteetti ja narratiivisuus*.
54. Lieblich et al., *Narrative Research*, 7–9.
55. Riessman, *Narrative Analysis*, 2.
56. Ibid., 5.
57. Lieblich et al. *Narrative Research*, 8.

differs from the community.⁵⁸ Ricoeur's distinction between sameness and selfhood is useful for this study because sameness gives tools to interpret otherness. Childlessness is interpreted as otherness in a community that stresses procreation. Selfhood is seen to be important in connection to the construction of strong self-esteem in spite of stigma of childlessness.

Holstein and Gubrium concentrate on narrative identity in a postmodern world. They claim that selves are constructed through storytelling. According to Holstein and Gubrium, narrative analysis centers on constructing identities and on the circumstances of narration.⁵⁹ The findings of Holstein and Gubrium reveal that as a method narrative analysis works well for studying identity. Narrative interpretations of identity stress the role of community in identity construction. This is a useful insight while studying identity construction in a communal Chagga context.

Analysis of the Data

Holistic-Content Analysis

The data in this study is analyzed in two ways: the narrative approach provides comprehensive views of complete narratives within holistic content analysis, and the Atlas-ti© software program provides effective categorical content analysis.⁶⁰ My theoretical position in the narrative theory comes very close to that of Lieblich, Tuval-Mashiach, and Zilber, and therefore I adopted two of their analysis strategies. The focus of my interest is on the content of the stories of childlessness. In order to focus on the content, I analyzed the content both holistically and categorically.⁶¹

Holistic content analysis is a method of reading and analyzing the life stories of subjects and focusing on their content. This requires reading the material many times, emphatically and with an open mind. Eventually some themes or topics are gleaned from the narratives. This kind of analytical method comes close to clinical case studies.⁶² When reading the narratives from my interviews using holistic content analysis, I recalled the interview situation and tried to form a holistic picture of the different couple's life stories.

The first step in handling the data was to convert the interviews into written form for later processing. All my tape-recorded narratives have

58. Ricoeur, *Oneself as Another*, 113–39.
59. Holstein and Gubrium, *Self We Live By*, 103–4.
60. Lieblich et al., *Narrative Research*, 12, 14, 163–64, 168–70.
61. See Ibid., 88–111, 141–64.
62. Ibid., 13, 62–63.

been transcribed in an electric form and the field notes are in a computer printout format in order to help my analysis. All interview tapes are saved in my collection. All rough transcriptions were done by Swahili-speaking research assistants, but the retranscriptions of the main narratives are mine. The interview data from the first phase was transcribed before the second phase took place. In the second phase of interviews each interview was transcribed as soon as it was conducted.

Riessman claims that transcriptions are both the beginning of the organizing process and the beginning of interpretation.[63] While doing the retranscriptions I got to know the narratives very well. Narrative analysis is a text-centered approach, and this means that the researcher has to concentrate on these texts. By transcribing carefully, interpretive categories emerge and ambiguities in language are heard on the tape. The way the story is told provides ready clues about its meaning.

An important part of this early stage of narrative analysis was the discussion about the research and processing the interviews. Narrative analysis is not only a matter of studying the narratives, but also to living and sharing them, as much as is possible, with the informants. Sharing the experience is as important as reading about the experience. This sharing was vital for in the final report and also during the process of analysis. I shared in such a way that the anonymity of interviewees was maintained at all times, discussing particular stories but not naming the individuals involved.

The actual analysis is a process of testing, clarifying, and deepening the understanding of what is happening in the narrative. Because narrative is the centre of holistic content analysis, I used analytic induction, which allows the questions to be modified when processing the narratives and also allows new questions to emerge. When interacting with the narratives, analytic ideas change.[64] Analytic induction was a valuable tool for interpreting the narratives in the present study, but it was not the only method of analysis used.

Holistic content analysis provided a tool to analyze the sample in order to find out how a childless couple constructs its identity. According to Lieblich et al., constructing of identity through autographical story and developing theory through empirical research are parallel processes.[65] Holistic content analysis provided the themes regarding how to organize my data into various categories.

63. Riessman, *Narrative Analysis*, 58.
64. Ibid., 60.
65. Lieblich et al. *Narrative Research*, 10.

Categorical Content Analysis

The data of this study was processed analytically after holistic content analysis had given a complete picture of the contents of a single interview. The analytical processing was done by using the Atlas-ti© software program for qualitative research.[66] Lieblich et al. term this type of analysis categorical content analysis, but it actually comes very close to traditional form of content analysis by searching for the deeper meanings of a certain text.[67]

There are two possible ways of using Atlas-ti© to code the data. The first is to develop codes from the empirical material. The second is to do the coding with a predefined code scheme. The reason for choosing this second option would be to link qualitative and quantitative analysis in later steps.[68] I preferred to use the first, more open, approach to code my narrative material. According to Kvale, coding narrative material mainly involves identifying themes in an individual narrative and constructing typologies from these themes.[69] When coding the narrative material, it is important to remember that the material is a part of a narrative and does not consist of autonomous elements that can be analyzed as such.

The process of categorical content analysis began with planning how to use the data in Atlas-ti©. I decided to have each separate interview as a "primary document," and after that decision was made, these primary documents were assigned to a "hermeneutic unit" in the program. Primary documents were grouped into "primary document families." I used the interview groups as primary document families, thus there were three separate families: church workers, parishioners, and childless persons. Locations were also used to group the interview data; thus, primary document families included both urban and rural parishes. Gender was used as further way to group the primary documents, so that male and female interviews could be dealt with separately.

All these primary documents were coded using loose coding categories. Some of the codes were created before the actual coding started based on the holistic content analysis, while others were created when a need arose to have a new category. Table 4 lists all the categories used and provides an idea as to what types of topics were included in each category. In the table there are also a total number of codes used in the whole sample. The total number of quotations was not listed to stress statistical treatment; rather, it was created in order to explore which topics emerged more often than others in the sample.

66. Flick, *Introduction*, 258.
67. Lieblich et al. *Narrative Research*, 112; Kvale, *Interviews*, 190–91.
68. Flick, *Introduction*, 259–60.
69. Kvale, *Interviews*, 190–91.

Table 4: Code Categories Used in Atlas-ti© Program

Code	Topics Included	Number of Quotations
Adoption	Adoption and fosterage	37
Coping	Various coping methods	53
Church teachings on marriage	Content and form of Lutheran church teachings on a Christian marriage	16
Family interference	The interference of mothers-in-law and other family members	15
Family secrets	Childlessness as a family secret	10
Guilt/shame	Situations of guilt and/or shame	15
Identity	Identity construction and comments on the identity of a childless person	31
Inheritance	Influence of childlessness on inheritance and stressing the importance of having a biological son	40
Insults	Lists of insults and their various interpretations	16
Search for help	Medical, spiritual, and traditional searches	43
Marriage counseling in the community	Counseling the couple in crisis by the family and neighborhood community	4
Polygyny	Polygyny as a traditional way to deal with childlessness	44
Practical hardships	Economic, social and spiritual hardships	26

Separation	Separation, desertion, and divorce	31
Singles in the community	Living single in the Chagga community, single mothers, and unofficial second wives	67
Staying together	All references to a committed union and reasons to stay together in spite of childlessness	6
Tension between Christian and traditional values/practices	Church discipline and burial practice	17
Traditional beliefs	Various beliefs connected to the burial of a childless person, sacrifices, and belief in witchcraft	22
Urban/rural	Interviewee analysis of the difference between lifestyle in a town and in a village	7

When doing the actual coding, direct quotations were marked. These quotations were used as condensed research data for later analyses. Codes were grouped into "code families," in which those codes that where similar to each other were grouped together. Since I had grouped the primary documents as families and codes as families, the Atlas-ti© program made it easy to search for separate outputs using various "selection criteria." This meant, for example, that if I wanted to extract quotations of male parishioners from the urban parish on polygyny, the program gave me this output.[70] A simple output of a one coding category was found to be very effective as well. For example, I used the output of all quotations about shame and guilt in the code when writing the section on shame and guilt in chapter 5. Another way to find exact information on the use of a single term was the use of word search function, which gave me a specific word and its use in all the primary documents. I used word search for specific Swahili terms to find out how the interviewees used and interpreted them.

70. Flick, *Introduction*, 259–60.

The Atlas-ti© program gives a further option of creating "memos" and "networks." I created some memos that contained my comments on the interpretation of a certain selected quotation. I found out, however, that it was more useful and attention grabbing to write these memos by hand on the printouts. I did use this feature of the program to create some networks that show connections between different codes and code families.

The combination of holistic content analysis and categorical content analysis provided me with the ideas for interpretation. The process of interpretation continued in beginnign to write the final report.

Interpretation of Narratives

Model Narratives—Typology versus Authentic Account

The interpretation of my interview data revealed three typical narratives of childless Chagga marriages. These model narratives have been selected and formulated carefully to represent the main types of life stories told during interviews. The decision to use model narratives instead of authentic personal stories was a difficult choice. It would have been much easier to use the authentic stories but I felt that it would not have been ethically proper. I did not want the interviewees, some of whom revealed their life secrets to an outsider for the first time, to suffer in the community because of their involvement in the research project. The final report, which uses model narratives, but which furthermore contains some authentic stories from interviews, works in a convincing way to narrate about the life of childless couples in Machame.

A danger of this approach is that model narratives might make the data of this study look too simple and coherent. I tried, however, to point to some of the naturally contradicting features in the model narratives. The model narratives of this study are not meant to be read as representative of all types of childless marriages. Using typology, in my case with model narratives, always gives a generalized result. My aim was to share some of the narratives with my reader in order to offer a better understanding of my theoretical analysis.

The data of this study consisted of both first- and third-person stories. Tremper Longman provides a helpful discussion of the differences between first- and third-person accounts. According to him, because the narrator in first-person stories is a character in the story, they present a limited point of view. Third-person stories refer to all the characters impersonally, since the narrator is usually an outsider in the story he/she tells.[71] In my data, many of the third-person narrators are not complete outsiders, but close relatives or friends of the childless couples, so their contribution to the communal interpretation of the life stories is considerable.

The final product of the study is model narratives that explain the experience of childlessness to the reader. When constructing these model narratives, I used both first-person and third-person stories. I analyzed the relationship of different narrators of the same story and compared the material I collected from each of them. The use of both first- and third-person narratives enables us to understand how people construct both personal and communal versions of the experience of childlessness.

There are, however, issues with the model stories because they were constructed using various first- and third-person descriptions. For example, in chapter 2, three original characters were used in the "Martha" narrative. One of the original "Marthas" of this story actually had a small baby after many childless years, and I could see how that influenced some of her comments. Another contradicting point in the same model narrative is that committed union includes a story of a "shortcut marriage," while some of the first-person narrators actually had a church wedding. Due to the necessity of coherence in narratives, in constructing the model narratives I had to leave out some individual experiences—even central ones—if they were not coherent to the plot of the model narrative. The unity of the three other model stories was easier to create because there was less material, and the material was not as diverse as in the first model narrative. Table 5 illustrates the sources from the research for the different model narratives.

My interpretation of the data was that the actors in these narratives resembled characters in the Old Testament. With that interpretation in mind, I ended up renaming the spouses of model narratives and generally used names from the Old Testament. For example, the women in the model narrative of desertion competed against one another for status, power, and a husband, not unlike Leah and Rachel in the biblical story, so I renamed these women after them, and named the husband Yakobo, the Swahili version of Jacob.

I did not, however, invite interpretation of these Old Testament stories during the interviews, and the result of this open-ended approach was that the narrators did not link their narratives to the biblical stories. Not a single first-person narrator linked her/his personal life experiences to

---

71. Longman, *Literary Approaches*, 85.

Table 5: Interviews Used to Construct Model Narratives

Model narrative	First-Person Interviews	Third-Person Interviews	Total Number of Interview Sources
Narrative of a committed union	4	5	9
Narrative of desertion	2	6	8
Narrative of official polygyny	3	3	6
Narrative of unofficial polygyny	2	1	3
Total	11	15	26

biblical stories, and only one third-person narrator made such a link on a general level.

The first model narrative is a story of committed union, which is presented and analyzed in chapter 2. This narrative was constructed using four first-person accounts, (among them the life story of an adopted son) and five third-person stories.

In chapter 4, two first-person life stories (one of a man and one of a woman) and six third-person interviews were used to create the model narrative of couple's crisis of childlessness that leads to the husband deserting his childless wife. The female first-person story dominates this narrative because she was interviewed twice, and her second, longer interview was tape-recorded. The male interview was not tape-recorded and his voice is only paraphrased in the model narrative, which makes his role less prominent.

In chapter 4, the data for the first model narrative of polygyny is mainly from third-person interviews; one elderly polygynous family was observed and interviewed briefly. Three third-person stories are used together with the first-person observation. The second model narrative, of unofficial polygyny, is constructed from two first-person interviews, one of an official wife and one of a concubine. I did not manage to meet the husband of the family. One third-person narrator gives her voice to explain more closely the family situation. During the field research I did not plan to use this narrative in my final report, therefore, I did not collect more third person narratives about it.

The use of twenty-six interviews to construct the four model narratives shows that more than half of the interviews in the sample of this study have been used to construct these narratives. Also, most of those interviews that did not contribute to the model narratives are used in chapters 5 and 6 for analyzing childlessness in Machame on a more abstract level.

Interpretation of narratives is always personal, partial, and dynamic. Interpretation requires dialogical listening, which is an interactive process with the narrative.[72] I certainly found that my own study was an interactive process with these life stories. I shared in the life stories of these interviewees during the whole process of this study, not only during the long field research period, but also during analysis and interpretation.

In narrative analysis it is important to open up interpretive issues for readers to see. The difficult issue of the power of the interpreter is always present. Riessman discusses the role of a narrative researcher and her/his influence on the final report.[73] I have struggled with this issue of power while writing the report for my study. I wonder, for example, what use is there in my research if the study is about narratives on childlessness in Kilimanjaro but the voice that is heard is the voice of a white, female foreigner who is not childless herself?

A further problem in evaluating my interpretations is that all my authentic stories are translations. In narrative analysis the reader usually has a possibility of checking the interpretation of the given narratives. I noted this problem from the beginning and tried to make as careful and literal translations as possible. However, English and Swahili are very different languages; consequently, in some parts I use the Swahili terminology to specify the terms used. All the direct stories in the final report are in English because many readers will not know Swahili. I have used a dynamic method of translation in order to grasp the main idea of people's stories. In order to condense and clarify the direct quotations, I have used several symbols to indicate how I have quoted the transliterated texts. I have used the following symbols:

---

72. Lieblich et al., *Narrative Research*, 10.
73. Riessman, *Narrative Analysis*, 61.

[. . .] Indicates that some words/names of places/sentences have been omitted either for safeguarding anonymity or avoiding repetition.

. . . Signifies a pause in the flow of speech.

(-) Indicates the addition of an explanatory word or phrase by the author.

[-] Indicates the addition of a missing word or phrase by the author.

In addition to using these symbols I omitted those comments of mine that did not add any meaning to the interview. Among these were exclamatory comments such as "Ehee!" or "Mhm!," sounds the polite listener makes in an African context.

Validity and Credibility of the Interpretation

Narrative analysis does not aim at numerical validity, but searches for a hermeneutical truth. This aim seeks to give the reader a hermeneutical experience that helps to see the world in a new light. Narrative analysis does not search for truth in order that such truth can be tested by empirical measures. Coherence in the narrative is a primary goal in narrative analysis. The question to be asked is not about what really happened but what the narrative reveals about a certain experience. The historical truth of an individual's life story was not the primary issue.[74] It is always possible to narrate the same events in radically different ways, as I have seen with my data, depending on the intent, values, and interests of the narrator.

The credibility in narrative research relies on good documentation of the oral material, and so tape-recording and proper field notes are important for the validity of narrative analysis. According to Donald Polkinghorne, when judging the credibility of a story we have to make a distinction between the accuracy of the data and the plausibility of the plot.[75] Narrative analysis is a text-centered approach, and there is a veto power of the text. It is not possible to write imaginary things if the researcher is bound to the text.[76]

Another aspect that we have to remember while judging the credibility of the life stories from Machame is that they were narrated in an official interview situation, in front of a tape recorder with a foreigner, though

---

74. Ibid., 64; Polkinghorne, *Narrative Configuration*, 21.
75. Polkinghorne, *Narrative Configuration*, 20.
76. Svartvik, *Mark and Mission*, 54–55.

usually the subject was previously acquainted with the interviewer. My presence and guiding questions certainly influenced the final narrative. If somebody else would have done these interviews in another situation, the final result of the life stories would be different. This does not mean, however, that the data used in this study is useless, rather, it means that we have to remember that it reveals only a part of the life story. Theoretical claims have to be supported with evidence from the informants' accounts, just as alternative interpretations of the data have to be considered.[77]

The Ethics of Research

Childlessness is a sensitive issue in Kilimanjaro. I had to struggle with ethnical decisions in all stages of the research process. After finding childless people willing to participate in the research, I had to ask them further whether I could record what was said. I felt hesitant as to whether it was ethically correct that I should make people talk in order to write a research paper. One childless person commented to me, "Why do you come to make me bleed again? Why have I to think again about those horrible years?" I did not have a ready answer for her questions, but when we continued to discuss her situation, she relaxed and found, ultimately, the interview had been therapeutic for her. She had not told her life story at such length before. While talking, she seemed to find inner meanings of her own life story and she learned that it is not always the best thing to be quiet about difficult experiences.

One method I used for keeping people's secrets was that, when I conducted interviews in homes, I always visited other homes in the same village. People in Kilimanjaro are very eager to gossip about their neighbors, and I did not want them to start gossiping about my interviewees. Some of the visits were normal pastoral visits to sick or elderly people in their homes or to meet some of the church elders of that village. Usually one of the homes I visited was where the actual interview took place.

Paying for the interviews would have been against my research ethic. I did not want to treat people as if they would be working for me. Paid workers want to please the employer and will try to give answers that they think the employer wants to hear. As I did not hire the interviewees, they were not bound by their comments. Some interviewees expected a payment after an interview, but did not demand it when I did not give them anything. Most of the interviewees did not expect anything from me. However, I wanted to thank some of those people who helped me

---

77. Riessman, *Narrative Analysis*, 61, 65–66.

frequently with a gift, for example, a new hymnbook. These were clearly gifts of thanks for their friendship, not payments for interviews. Gifts were also given to me; many times I returned home with bananas or fresh maize for my children.

A difficult part of the research process was when I the field after a long period of contact. I had grown so used to visiting these people regularly and I felt empty without regular contact with them. I slowly started to prepare members of the study communities for the fact that I was leaving.

While analyzing the data, I struggled for a long time with a dilemma: Should I involve the subjects of this study in the interpretation or not? Interviewees did not ask for these interpretations and I decided not to include them, but I did include other insiders who gave feedback. These insiders were not included in the sample of the study, but they could, however, give valuable feedback to my interpretations. Dr. Fredrik Shoo, the Machame-born bishop of the Northern Diocese, read chapters 2–4 and gave his valuable comments and corrections to my interpretations. Regular discussions with my Chagga colleagues, Rev. Zakayo I. Kimaro and Rev. Emeline Ndossi, helped me improve my interpretations as well. Another reason that contributed to my decision to leave the subjects out of the feedback process was that the interpretations are done from the constructed model narratives and would not contain analysis on any one individual. The final struggle had to do with maintaining confidentiality in reporting. I left out some central authentic accounts in order to safeguard the interviewees. My goal was that nobody who shared their experiences with me would encounter any problems because they were involved in my research process.

2

Narrative of a Committed Union

Official Marital Form Was Important

THE FOCUS OF THIS chapter is to analyze the coping strategies of an infertile couple that helped the couple to stay together. The narrative of Martha and Yeremia illustrates the marital life of a committed couple in Machame.

Martha is thought to be a very beautiful Chagga woman. She has "fair" skin and, in Machame where many are quite dark skinned, this is a highly valued characteristic in women. Martha finished her primary education and afterwards stayed on her parents' farm. Yeremia is an educated man. Before getting married twenty years ago, Yeremia was teaching at the local primary school. Martha was twenty years old, and Yeremia some years older, when they moved together into Yeremia's small rented room in a suburban area outside of Moshi. Martha explains the beginning of their marriage:

MARTHA: *At that time when I got married this way. My father came . . . He told my partner, if you married my child I want your signature. O.K., my husband wrote his signature and I wrote my signature and after this I remained with him. Fine, after this I stayed with my husband here in X (name of place omitted) since we had our marriage officiated. At that time the pastor got a transfer and he told us that he cannot leave his friends outside of the parish and then he took us back to the parish and blessed our marriage. [. . .] At that time didn't he sign in front of my father? And he did sign again in front of the church, how could he divorce me?*

The explanation of the signatures was very important for Martha. The signatures pointed to the marital security and to the official form of their marriage. Martha's selection of words is interesting. In the beginning of her story she calls him "partner," but she calls him "husband" only after the official signatures. On another occasion she replied by using the same words: "He had signed and I had signed so we were officially married." She denies the possibility of divorce but the fact that she mentions it shows that she or the surrounding community had considered it as a possibility. Martha is not a verbally gifted person and could not reason any more on her comment.

Marriage in a patriarchal Chagga community is a bond between two families. Because of this, couples like Martha and Yeremia, who used a "shortcut marriage," that is, they lived together, usually discuss their marriage with both families. Martha only mentioned her father's visit, but most likely there were other discussions with Yeremia's family as well. What seems to be missing from Martha's narrative is the discussion of her bride wealth. Perhaps transactions of the normal bride wealth were not included, and this made the signature the only sign of an official union. Usually in these "shortcut marriages," some bride wealth may be paid later on. In Chagga society the bride wealth connects the two families together. None of the narratives revealed any negative attitude towards bride wealth. It seems that most of the time bride wealth continues to be an important connection between the two families and helps sustain marriages in Machame.

Martha speaks in a very natural way about the time when they were under church discipline. This does take up a large portion of Martha's narrative, for she considers her official marital bond more important than a church wedding. She experienced the support of her natal family in her marital agreement. Martha narrates how the pastor of the urban parish received a transfer to another parish and did not want to leave Martha and Yeremia under church discipline, so he blessed their marriage in the church before he left. The pastor in Martha's narrative is described as a friend who cared for their marriage. Martha does not stress the penal nature of church discipline; the hospitable attitude of the pastor is more central in her story.

The official marital tie, as revealed in Martha's central narrative, helped Martha and Yeremia during the early years of their marriage. Because they had not had a child, they could not live without some family interference in a community that expects a child to be born soon in every marriage.

Insults Were Finished after a Family Meeting

Martha and Yeremia had been married for three years and without any signs of having a child. The young couple continued to live in a suburban area quite far from Yeremia's family. Martha and Yeremia did not live with his in-laws, a fact which Martha emphasized several times. She even pointed out how they lived in the suburban village and her in-laws were ten kilometers away. They were clearly not within hearing distance. While commenting on the geographical distance, Martha pointed to two things: firstly, she emphasized the fact that from their home to her in-laws was quite a long distance and it would be impossible to shout loudly enough for the in-laws to hear; secondly, she pointed to the psychological distance between them, which meant that the family could not interfere in their everyday life because they lived so far away.

Psychological distance seems to indicate a growing independence from Yeremia's family. Traditional Chagga families are not only patriarchal but also patrilocal. In an urban situation, as is the case with Martha and Yeremia, young couples have more independence than if they lived in his parents' homestead.

Martha narrated how she had a good relationship with her mother-in-law, but not so with all Yeremia's relatives. The sisters-in-law were eager to insult Martha because of her childlessness. Martha told a story about these insults:

AULI: *We discussed how people talk badly . . .*

MARTHA: *Yes, these things are there, words exist.*

AULI: *And what do you think, why do they say in such a way?*

MARTHA: *For that time when you live in that home and they see that you are not from there, these words have to appear.*

AULI: *So they see that the work of a wife is to give birth?*

MARTHA: *Yes.*

AULI: *So it is not only a joy to find a spouse for their child but it is also important to reproduce . . .*

MARTHA: *They are happy but anyhow she should give birth.*

AULI: *So these two things go together?*

MARTHA: *Yes.*

Martha's way of talking about the insults surprised me. I wanted to know more about them and how she felt about them. Martha explained about thyem casually, as if they were not something amazing, as it was for me at that stage. From her story we see that her interpretation is that the insults are natural, something that have to come because a wife is expected to give birth.

Third-person narrators explained the contents of the insults. Martha generally agreed that these harsh words were spoken but did not want to recall them. The insulters told Martha face-to-face that the work of a wife is to give birth. They continued insulting her by saying that she is eating food for nothing. Yeremia heard insults such as "What is the use of a wife who does not give birth?" and "Did he marry her just to fill the toilet?" Neither Martha nor Yeremia recalled these insults themselves. Recalling the exact insults seemed hard on Martha, and she admitted that there had been such words but did not want to recall them. Martha additionally recalls that Yeremia was advised to take another wife or to have a child outside of marriage. However, she agreed that those who spoke such words had a reason to do so; a child is a must in a Chagga marriage.

One sister of Yeremia was more active than the others in insulting Martha. Yeremia contacted his sister and explained how he had married Martha and how God had given Martha to him to be his partner, and, even if they did not have children, they wanted to continue to live together. This episode, which was narrated by another sister of Yeremia, includes Yeremia's confession of his love for Martha. This small story is interesting in that it reveals the companionship and unity of Martha and Yeremia. They continued to be dependent on each other. A Chagga man himself would probably not have mentioned such an intimate comment. Still, based on the life of Martha and Yeremia, it seems that this third-person interpretation might come quite close to Yeremia's ideas.

Martha and Yeremia decided to have a family meeting to put an end to these insults and put an end to the advice given to Yeremia that he should father children outside of their marriage. Martha explains how difficult this time was for them:

MARTHA: *I and my husband we waited (for a child) in peace but there outside words appeared.*

AULI: *Were these words outside your home?*

MARTHA: *Yes, from outside.*

AULI: *Were they from family or only from neighbors?*

MARTHA: *From family, yes, sisters-in-law. Words appeared but we silenced these words.*

AULI: *What would you say: Did you have to answer to these insults or did you stay silent if you heard them or did they talk more to your husband?*

MARTHA: *They talked maybe to my husband but we interfered and that was the end of these insults.*

Martha's narrative of the family meeting is another central part of her life story. It again reveals the companionship of the young couple. Martha tells that they, as a young couple, organized the meeting and many members of the family were present. In a Chagga context, it is very atypical for a young couple to organize a family meeting themselves. A more natural way would be for them to see an elder of the clan and ask him to set up such a meeting. Martha does not clearly indicate in her story how this meeting was organized. It is, however, seen that the spouses planned the meeting together. The narrative of the family meeting reveals the sympathetic nature of the marital and communal support given to Martha and Yeremia, but it also reveals a growing independence from his family's coercion.

Martha's narrative of the family meeting suggests there is a high degree of gender equality in marriage and social position possible in Machame, where women have better educational opportunities and more bargaining power in marriage than in some other societies in Tanzania. Martha herself is not an educated person, but Yeremia's education seems to have contributed to increased gender equality in their marriage. Another important factor that seemed to make their marriage cooperative was that they both had a good sense of self-esteem.

After the family meeting, the insults stopped, except from the main contributor, Yeremia's elder sister. The third-person narrator stresses that even today Yeremia and Martha are not in regular contact with her. As years passed, Martha and Yeremia's marriage transitioned from its cooperative state to a period of years of searching for the reason for their infertility problem.

Years of Crisis

It is common knowledge in the neighborhood that Martha and Yeremia have an infertility problem, but there are very few people who have heard them discuss it. One of the pastors took the initiative and visited Martha and Yeremia. She explained that the church worker has to be active in this type of case because a childless couple may feel lonely and society may them. Another third-person narrator explained how this pastor and some of the church elders went to Martha and Yeremia's home to visit them and pray on their behalf. One of the elders received a prophecy during the prayer, which revealed that Martha and Yeremia would have a child in a year.

Two years passed and there were still no signs of a child. When the prophecy did not come true, Yeremia felt depressed. The following account is from a transcribed interview with the female pastor in the urban parish:

PASTOR: *I asked him, how does he feel? He explained how badly he feels. All these years he stayed with his wife and they had not managed to get a child. And that one replied, really on that day he said, "I would be ready to kill myself now." [. . .]*

AULI: *It seems that he really felt bad.*

PASTOR: *He felt as . . . It would be better I would leave this world. He said: "It would be better I go to the Father."*

The above discussion illustrates how depressed Yeremia felt after the failed prophecy. This suggests that the physical problem hindering conception is more on Yeremia's side. There seems to be general conclusion in their neighborhood that Yeremia has the physical problem, but this was never said during any of the official interviews. This avoidance of commenting on Yeremia's infertility is because, traditionally, only women are understood to be infertile in the Chagga context. A childless person, or *tasa*, is always a woman. A man cannot be *tasa*; he is referred to as somebody who does not have the male capacity or power.[1] It is a very strong comment, and the interviewees used it only with regard to general comments on male infertility. It would be an insult to direct this comment at a specific person; it actually means that a person is impotent in all ways, not just that he does not have children. Infertility is a threat to men and nullifies proof of their virility and masculine procreativity.[2]

Usually the blame for childlessness falls to the woman, even in cases like Martha and Yeremia's where the cause seems to be on husband's side. Most of the time men are protected from blame by patriarchal ideology. Chagga men want to feel prestige for their manhood, and many of them are not prepared to go to a hospital for a medical checkup.

The same female pastor of the urban parish continued to explain why a pastor has to take an active role in such cases. This short explanation followed the previous one in her interview. She was still explaining more about her visit to Martha and Yeremia's home. Her aim was to explain how pastoral counseling towards childless couples should be organized:

---

1. See also Mgalla and Boerma, "Discourse of Infertility," 191.
2. See also Inhorn, *Infertility and Patriarchy*, 12, 63; Riessman, "Even If We Don't Have Children," 135.

PASTOR: *It is until a pastor is ready to go and visit them.*

AULI: *Mhm. Yes, so they do not come to you?*

PASTOR: *They will not come to you.*

AULI: *To ask from you?*

PASTOR: *No, they will not come to you.*

AULI: *Is it the work of a pastor to seek them?*

PASTOR: *To seek them. Because they feel lonely, they feel desperate here, and, in addition to that, the society may have neglected them. Because of this they seek help from a person who seeks them. Neither person who . . . They are not themselves those who seek help. They cannot go. You have to build friendship with them and only after that they will come to you.*

Pastors in both study parishes felt that it was difficult to approach the committed, childless couples. These couples do not talk openly about their problem but want to keep their childlessness as a secret. After coming to know a pastor better, they can open to her or him.

The narrative of Martha and Yeremia does not reveal whether they went for medical checkups. Martha mentions in her life story only that she did not use birth control pills before her marriage. The following account discusses Martha's attitude towards birth control and abortion.

MARTHA: *I had a good relationship with my mother-in-law and did not use birth control pills. [. . .]*

MARTHA: *Others do abortions, do you know?*

AULI: *Yes.*

MARTHA: *If she does an abortion, you will see in which way God took care of you. So you will not get children even later.*

AULI: *And what do you think? Are abortions common nowadays? Are they done many times?*

MARTHA: *Many times, girls make a lot of abortions. God gave you one or two eggs or you find that God gave only one creature in your stomach and while aborting you lose that. And they go to make abortion! They are them who have problems with their husbands.*

The Chagga community expects that a child will be born as soon as possible, and because of this it is understood that contraceptives are used only for premarital sex or after a certain number of children are born.

It is important for Martha's self-esteem that she did not have premarital sexual relationships. She asserts that pills and other modern things are bad. Martha seems to share the widespread belief across African continent that the use of contraceptives causes infertility.[3]

Martha continues, after a short personal comment, on a separate explanation regarding the reasons for infertility. She points to young girls, to the next generation, and how they do all kinds of bad things. She maintains that these young girls have abortions. Abortion is illegal in Tanzania, but they are performed either at hospitals by bribing officials or by unofficial abortionists.[4] Martha came to the conclusion that if somebody has an abortion God will not give that person a child. Her biological explanation was that if God gave a certain girl one or two eggs and she has an abortion, no egg is left after the abortion.[5]

In her narrative, Martha does not consider the possibility of male infertility while she points to those girls who have abortions. She seems to share the cultural point of view that infertility is a female problem. It seems that with this narrative, Martha wants to show how she differs from these girls. She is a respected wife whose husband does not cause her problems. Martha did not have any issues to be reconciled and this gave her a strong sense of self-esteem. Martha does not reveal whether she knew the reason as to why they do not have a child; at least she does not discuss it in her narrative.

Gradually Martha and Yeremia learned to live without a child and many people started to see them as a harmonious couple. They like each other and cope well together and have not lost their hope. They respect each other and do not compete with each other. Neighbors seem to praise them, especially Yeremia, about how good a husband he is to not to marry a second wife or show anger towards his wife. The conclusion is that God has helped Martha and Yeremia to stay peacefully together. Two separate explanations from the same third-person narrator reflect this good relationship between the spouses. These accounts are told in two different interviews, and both praise Martha and Yeremia's committed marital union.

PARISHIONER: *The husband of that woman, he is committed to his wife; he does not lose his patience. Because you see that he does not take another wife, nor show his disrespect to his wife. They both stay committed, they stay committed. Even though husband has to listen to the blames of his parents still he does not lose his patience nor show disrespect.*

3. Mgalla and Boerma, "Discourse of Infertility," 194.
4. See also Hasu, *Desire and Death*, 345–49.
5. See also Mgalla and Boerma, "Discourse of Infertility," 191.

Another account from this same female parishioner, which is in her later interview, explains their relationship even more. This account is unusual for the way it openly explains the love of Yeremia to Martha. In a Chagga context, the word love is not regularly used; the idea is mainly discussed using other words such as "they have good cooperation."

PARISHIONER: *They stay committed and they love each other. They share their thoughts together. They have not lost their hope. And they are people who fear God. [. . .] One thing that they do is that they communicate well. Neither one is tired of the other spouse. They do not live in order to compete against each other.*

An important term, which is repeated many times during the interviews, is *kuvumilia*, to have patience or to tolerate. This is especially connected to the case of Martha and Yeremia. People see that this couple live peacefully together; they cope well with the stress of being childless and they respect and fear God. From the Chagga cultural point of view, to openly react to a problem shows a lack of maturity. Martha and Yeremia have now entered their thirties, and in their adult relationship urgent pressures for a child have become more visible.

Decision to Adopt a Son

Martha and Yeremia like children, and neighbors recall that they actively play with the children who visit them. As time passed it was not enough for Martha and Yeremia merely to have children visit them, and they started worrying as to who would inherit their house and farm after their deaths. They needed to have a child, preferably a son, who would also take care of them when they are old.

Martha and Yeremia started to search for a child. They did not want a child of a relative to be raised in their house, but they wanted to have a small orphan who would not belong to any family. They found young Eliezer, whose mother had died when giving birth to him. Eliezer's mother had been single and there were no demands from her family to keep the child. After the death of his mother, Eliezer stayed in the hospital orphanage waiting to eventually move somewhere else. Martha and Yeremia adopted Eliezer and raised him as their own son.

Martha and Yeremia were happy with Eliezer and did their best to take care of him and to educate him. Some neighbors discuss why Martha and Yeremia did not take a child from the family, as is more common among the Chagga. One friend thought it would have been better had they fostered a child of a brother, as the child would be a relative. Another person felt that adoption would be a better option. A foster child is often too old to get used to a new home.

The cultural reason for preferring adoption to fosterage was explained to me. In the Chagga community, fostered children of a relative are often given the status of domestic servants; girls are used to help with the work in the house while boys take care of the domestic animals. According to the third-person narrator, an adopted child is seen to be more neutral, not related to either of the spouses, as would be the case of a foster child. Legal adoption is very rare in Kilimanjaro as in other parts of Tanzania. Kayongo-Male and Onyango claim that the reluctance to adopt children legally shows that adopted children are not an acceptable solution to a problem of childlessness in Africa.[6]

Eliezer was quite old when he got to know the family of his biological mother. He recalls this in an interview the first time when he went to visit his mother's family on the other side of Machame. His blood relatives wanted him to return home, but Eliezer did not want to leave Martha and Yeremia who had taken care of him and whom he considered as his parents. Eliezer had grown with Martha and Yeremia and could not think of leaving them. Without Eliezer's support, the approaching of old age for Martha and Yeremia would be much harder. Now they had a son who will take care of their physical and psychological needs.

Adoption was a solution for the infertility crisis of Martha and Yeremia. Their decision to go with formal adoption might still result in some difficulties later on. Narratives on adoption in both study parishes reveal that adoption is understood to be a problematic coping strategy in a Chagga context. The problem is that an adopted child is not a blood relative. Blood is an important connection to land in Machame. Only a male child can inherit the ancestral land around a Chagga homestead. The family graves are on this land, which makes it a special place. The other land, in this case lowland farms, is normal property and not considered special.[7]

One of the pastors explained why a biological child is so important. He maintained that an adopted son cannot conduct the traditional sacrifices after the death of his parents because the family forefathers are not present. This pastor is the only one I heard speak openly about sacrifices to ancestors; however, this reason seemed to explain other people's preference for fosterage as opposed to adoption. Others pointed out that the sacrifices

---

6. Kanyongo-Male and Onyango, *Sociology*, 106.
7. Stambach, *Lessons*; Hasu, *Desire and Death*, 478–83.

are sometimes done secretly, but this pastor explained very openly how adoption is made difficult because of these rituals.

In order to understand the above discussion regarding the stress on having a biological child, we have to explore the Chagga conception of life after death. According to Aaron Urio, the Chagga in their traditional religion make no attempt to distinguish between the physical and the spiritual world. In connection to life after death, various rituals are important in order to secure immortality for a deceased person. These require rituals, many of which are still practiced today, and which can only be performed by their blood descendants. Urio asserts further that without procreation one was considered completely cut off from the family, both in this life and in the hereafter. Childlessness was thus considered an absolute death.[8]

The stress on biological continuity, which I believe derives from the African understanding of immortality, is clearly seen in third-person comments in connection to the adoption of Eliezer. Fosterage of children is common in a Chagga context, but it is always understood that these children each belong to their biological father's clan and will keep their father's name in spite of the fact that they have been raised somewhere else. African immortality stresses the need to have a child in order to continue living after the earthly life and in order to be remembered by the family and by the larger community. Behind the stress on African immortality, there seems to be an understanding of life as a vital force that is passed on from parents to their child and later to their grandchildren.[9] Life comes from the physical parent and this is what makes adoption impossible for those who follow the traditional thinking. The continuation of life is central and should not be cut off for any reason.

One way the departed are remembered is by naming children after them. Normally a child is named after a grandparent in order for the departed to remain an influential member of the living community. The first name can be just a given name, but many times nowadays the second name of a person is the name of a grandparent. The first son will get a name of his paternal grandfather and the second son the name of his maternal grandfather. Similarly, daughters will be named after their grandmothers.[10] The naming of Eliezer differs from this procedure. Martha and Yeremia decided to give him a biblical name that is not used in their families. They did not give him a second name that would show connection to the paternal family, as would normally be the tradition with the firstborn

---

8. Urio, *Concept of Memory*, 105–9, 119.
9. Tempels, *La philosophie bantoue*, 41–44.
10. Urio, *Concept of Memory*, 118–19; Shoo, "Traditional African Marriage," 25.

son. Martha and Yeremia indicated when choosing Eliezer's name that the Christian cultural category better suits the situation of adoption. Carrying the name of a grandparent indicates that a child's life comes from there, but in a case of adoption, following the Chagga tradition for naming is not possible.

The narrative of Martha and Yeremia does not reveal how inheritance will work in Eliezer's case. Martha and Yeremia are a now a middle-aged couple and their son is a young adult. The discussion about the importance of being a blood relative shows once more, however, the strong patriarchal nature of the Chagga community in Machame, and sheds more light on the intense pressure of paternity on Chagga men.[11]

Identities of Adoption Parents

The adoption of Eliezer took place many years ago. Family and neighbors are now used to the idea of adoption and narrate concerning the parental identities of this committed couple. One third-person account explains that Martha is an active member of the women's group at her local Lutheran church. The patriarchal community does not pressure Martha any longer, perhaps because it seems that she has a strong identity. The explanation of her role in the church community reveals her strong self-esteem:

PARISHIONER: *She is active and likes to attend.*

AULI: *All right, so it does not give her problems even if . . .*

PARISHIONER: *She does not have any problems.*

AULI: *So, it does not give her problems to join other women at the church even though she does not have a child herself?*

PARISHIONER: *It does not bring any problems. [. . .] She is cheerful, completely happy when you see her. Her situation is just as you saw it. [. . .] One cannot see that she would be depressed. She got used to being childless. She exists, exists, and fits well in the group. She has not taken it as a stigma or invalidity. She sees it is alright. [. . .] She is even the chairperson of our group. And the meaning is that she is a very organized woman. (Swahili language calls her mother, but the meaning is a woman or a wife.) She is an organized and lively person. She likes to cooperate with others. And she has love and all other good qualities. She has a good reputation.*

---

11. Compare to the findings of Inhorn, *Infertility and Patriarchy*, 13.

The above account reveals that Martha does not have any problems attending the meetings at the church. A neighbor woman praises Martha with many words. This third-person narrator refers to Martha, however, as a childless woman, in spite of the fact that Eliezer was already adopted. However, it should be noted that while asking the questions in this interview I myself defined Martha as being childless, as I did not yet know at that time about the adoption of a child.

Adoption has made Martha a social mother, but she will remain biologically childless for the rest of her life in the eyes of her neighborhood. In discussing the issues of raising children, she shares her experience with other women in the church. The rest of the community sees that she lacks a biological child who can inherit the characteristics of his/her parents, Yeremia's family name, and, rightfully, inherit the family farm.

It seems from this narrative that in this particular women's group Martha has found her own place in the community. Motherhood does not seem to be the most central part of Martha's social identity. Martha is an active woman and capable of being a leader of the women's group. This seems to indicate that she does not construct her identity only from motherhood, but from other aspects such as her dairy projects, which helps her to build strong self-esteem as a respected member of the community.

The role of an adopted father seems to be more difficult for Yeremia, yet he is very proud of Eliezer and in an informal discussion explained about his plans for Eliezer's future studies. Infertility is a serious blemish on a man's social identity in Machame, but Yeremia is willing to look for new models and new way of understanding fatherhood. Fatherhood has traditionally been central in constructing the identity of a man in Kilimanjaro. It has been so important in a traditional Chagga society that a male relative of a barren husband would father a child with the barren man's wife in order to release him from the shame of infertility. In the contemporary community this does not seem to be that common. It seems to be more common that committed wives like Martha cope with their husband's suspected infertility.

Yeremia does not construct his male identity based only on his relationship with Eliezer. Rather, career seems to be central for Yeremia's identity. Yeremia has proceeded with his teaching career and currently he is the principal of one of the colleges in the area. Now at the peak of his career, he is very proud of his farm and the big brick house he has managed to build. Yeremia is well-educated, financially well-off, and a valued member of his home parish and the neighborhood community. He is also an active parishioner who has served as a church elder in the urban parish.

The relationship between Yeremia and Martha seems to function well. They have both found their respective gender identities as adoptive parents in the community and their behavior reveals that they both have strong self-esteem. After the years of crisis, it appears that Martha and Yeremia have a committed union and their adoption of Eliezer sustains their marriage.

Holy Wedlock?

Many Christians, including Lutherans, use the Swahili term *ndoa takatifu*, holy wedlock, when describing a Christian marriage. *Ndoa takatifu* is connected especially to marriages officiated in the church, but also to those infertile marriages that are stable, as in case of Martha and Yeremia. Unlike the stories of other couples who have a committed union, Martha and Yeremia did not have a church wedding. Many third-person accounts stress the importance of the church wedding for a successful marital union in the midst of infertility. Martha and Yeremia's narrative supports the idea of a committed union even though the couple used the common "shortcut marriage." It shows that the society and also the church gladly accept these types of marriages which are later blessed in the church.

The data of this research reveals that marital issues are widely discussed in both of the parishes studied. All interview groups commented on church teachings with regard to marriage. Many of the parishioners explained the type of seminars available in their parish. Workers included explanations of the contents of these courses, and the teaching about marriage was for couples before the wedding.

The narrative of Martha and Yeremia reveals many important factors that could help an infertile Chagga couple to avoid the common collapse of infertile marriages. It narrates the marital life of an infertile couple in urban Kilimanjaro. The African family interferes with the situation, but this does not need to affect the marital life as it might do in a rural setting, where the young couple lives in the same homestead as the husband's in-laws. Jackson Malewo claims that a spousal relationship controlled by the parents and other in-laws cannot grow in an African context.[12]

This particular model narrative reveals good communal support from both sides of the families. The texts are fairly sparse, but they reveal an understanding of Martha's father's concern over his daughter's marriage during his visit to the young couple and again at the family meeting that ended the insults. This shows the family support for Martha and Yeremia.

---

12. Malewo, *Pre-marital Counseling*, 44.

The parish community was also concerned with their marital life. The visits of the pastor and church elders showed Martha and Yeremia that they were not left outside the faith community and that there were people who were concerned that they might be feeling lonely or isolated.

The model narrative of a committed union also points to other important factors for sustaining an infertile marriage in Chagga society. The pressure of paternity is very strong on Chagga men. In those cases where the physical problem is on the side of the wife, many Chagga men end up seeking a child out of wedlock. In those cases where the actual problem is on husband's side, the Chagga man has to learn to cope with his infertility. Marcia Inhorn had similar findings in her study among poor urban Egyptians. She writes how women are expected to cope with childlessness and stay in their marriage even when the infertility problem is attributed to the husband.[13]

The case of Martha and Yeremia is a good example of a couple keeping a family secret even though everybody seems to know their secret, but very few people would admit that they would have discussed the problem with them. Infertility, especially suspected male infertility, is a family secret and as such is not discussed openly in the Chagga community. If a man is unable to father children it is understood to be very shameful and thus male infertility is a kept a secret. The infertile status of men is not disclosed. Only the closest relatives will know the truth of male infertility.[14]

Other factors clearly seen in our model narrative that may lead to more stable marriages are higher education and a sound financial situation.[15] Well-off families have a better chance of coping with childlessness, although such couples still feel a need to have a child. These couples do not have as great a need for child labor as in the case of poor peasant families.

Martha and Yeremia used adoption as their strategy to cope with childlessness. Adoption shows how modern a couple they are, as official adoptions are still very rare in Kilimanjaro. Mgalla and Boerma found in their research that only the younger respondents mentioned adoption as a coping strategy in infertile Sukuma marriages.[16] Fostering a child of a relative remains a more common way to cope with childlessness. Martha and Yeremia have remained married despite the disappointment of infertility and the social stigma of childlessness. The following chapter discusses a narrative in which the crisis of infertility leads to marital collapse.

13. Inhorn, *Infertility and Patriarchy*, 123.
14. Mgalla and Boerma, "Discourse of Infertility," 196.
15. Inhorn, *Infertility and Patriarchy*, 125.
16. Mgalla and Boerma, "Discourse of Infertility," 197–98.

3

Narrative of Desertion

The Early Years of an Infertile Marriage

THIS CHAPTER FOCUSES ON the crisis of infertility leading to marital separation. The narrative of Leah and Yakobo provides a lens to explore how infertility affects a couple—the man, the woman, and their relationship. When exploring the effects on a couple, both spouses are also studied individually. The individual study focuses on seeing how a middle-aged woman works to cope with her childlessness and to construct a positive identity while also examing how the pressure of a patriarchal society affects the life and self-esteem of a Chagga man.

Leah lives in a Chagga community where women are expected to marry and bear children. She is in her late forties. She was married at less than twenty years of age to Yakobo, who was from her home village in Kilimanjaro. She came from a poor home with many children. Her father had been sick for many years and this deeply influenced the financial situation of her family, as all their income was used for her father's medical care. During the time of interviews, Leah had been separated from Yakobo for a long time. He is the first-born son in his family, and has been working most of his adult life outside his home village as a government official.

Leah described the early years of her marriage as happy. The relationship between the spouses was good and they lived happily together. Yakobo was working away from home in different Tanzanian towns like many other young men from the village. Leah visited him sometimes but she mainly stayed on his farm in the village and took care of animals and the fields. Leah described this time as having been harmonious and full of work.

Leah emphasized the importance of farming for her identity during these years. When explaining about her agricultural tasks, Leah seemed to stress that she was a respected farmer, not somebody who was living a lazy life without work. Straight after the story on farming, Leah turned to discuss her girlhood life.[1] She seemed to stress her respectable role while telling these two explanations, one after the other:

LEAH: *I took care of my virginity from childhood until I was married. This helped me a lot. There was not blame, such as I do not know if you did that and that, if you have gone with men. That is the reason why you do not have a child. Maybe you had an abortion!*

AULI: *And your husband knew this?*

LEAH: *Eee! Yes he . . .*

AULI: *That you had a good reputation?*

LEAH: *Yes this was the most important thing, that when I got married I had not done anything. [. . .] It helped me to respect myself, even if somebody did not want to believe me, it helped me. [. . .] So to take care of your girlhood helps a lot, you cannot get blamed at any way. And even . . . I in my marriage did not complain.*

While explaining the early years of her marriage Leah stressed how she took care of herself before the marriage. This is an important topic to which she returned many times while telling about her youth. She was very young at the time of her marriage and did not have premarital sexual relationships. She discussed how some girls have abortions and, because of this, do not have children. She maintained in her narrative that she herself did not do anything wrong. Leah shares the common understanding in Africa that contraceptive use leads to infertility.

Important in the early years of Yakobo and Leah's marriage was the visible lack of a child. Years went by and there was no sign of a child. In the following account, Leah narrates this time of their marriage:

LEAH: *The time went on and I did not get a child [. . .] I tried to live this way . . . but we did not quarrel neither provoke each other, not even a little, until we had been married for about six years. During the seventh year he started to see that . . . he saw that there was no child . . .*

In spite of the lack of a child, Leah recalled this time as harmonious. Yakobo coped well with childlessness in the beginning. But Leah's story reveals that Yakobo later became quite depressed over not having a child in his marriage. In story two, Leah does not narrate about the medical examinations, but in another interview, which was not tape-recorded, she explained her medical examinations in a local hospital. She went to see a

---

1. Bülow, "Power, Prestige," 12; Howard and Millard, *Hunger and Shame*, 146–47.

doctor who told her to wait. She stressed that the doctor did not find anything to be wrong with her and told here that she should just wait. Leah did not use much time to describe whether there were any infertility treatments and did not name where she went for her checkup. Her purpose in this part of her life story was to stress that the doctor found there was nothing wrong with her. Leah explained that the doctor interpreted the reason for infertility to be the absence of Yakobo; the young couple met too seldom and this was the reason Leah did not conceive.

This part of Leah's life story suggests self-assurance. She does not blame herself for infertility. She ded not concentrate on infertility checkups in her narrative. Most central is that she was checked and nothing was found to be wrong with her.[2] Leah purported that the reason for her misfortune was not something she had done. Leah did not reveal in her narrative if any attempts of reconciliation were made because of the infertility, or if some sacrifices were made for the ancestors. The traditional Chagga understanding is that misfortune is somebody's fault and through reconciliation wholeness can be restored.

Leah said the harmonious time of her marriage lasted about six years, but then her parents-in-law started to interfere with the life of the young couple by asking what the problem was. This family interference was very hard for Leah. Leah and Yakobo stayed together for a rather long period for being in a culture that stresses procreation. There was, however, a change to come in their relationship: Yakobo lost hope of having a child in his marriage with Leah.

Family Advises the Husband to Desert His Wife

Leah lived together with her in-laws and this made her life hard.[3] Her mother-in-law and sisters-in-law both gave Leah a hard time. Leah recalled how others in the same homestead lived a good life whereas she had financial difficulties. Many times she thought things might be different if she would have had a child. The following account of Leah describes the family interference in their marriage:

LEAH: *I did not have any problems, except from his parents. They asked why their son has not got a child. They asked what the problem is. They wanted to know the reason and that hurt a lot, pastor . . .*

AULI: *Did both of them comment so?*

---

2. Inhorn, *Infertility and Patriarchy*, 117; Riessman, "Personal Troubles," 79.
3. Kafunzile, "Shame and Its Effects," 104; Inhorn, *Infertility and Patriarchy*, 125, 171–76.

LEAH: *Mother-in-law, mother-in-law and her daughters. [. . .]*

AULI: *And from the side of your family?*

LEAH: *My family . . .*

AULI: *They did not see a problem?*

LEAH: *They did, but now you know, they carried my burden as their own.*

The behavior of Leah's in-laws shows the strong patriarchal nature of family structure in Machame, where women are famous for being difficult mothers-in-law. In many parts of Kilimanjaro, the Machame women are called *wapalestina*, the Palestinians, because they are so eager to fight.[4]

Leah recalled her situation as being financially difficult. Yakobo did not support his official wife any longer. Many times when coming to visit his home village, he went to see only his mother and father and did not come to see Leah. During the two interviews, Leah frequently stressed her lack of financial support in the different stages during her life story. In the Chagga culture, giving gifts is a way of showing that one really cares. The lack of financial support on the part of her husband showed Leah, even before the actual desertion, that Yakobo did not care about her any longer.

The relationship between Leah and her in-laws is a typical situation in a patriarchal society where women compete with each other for power. Women's power increases with seniority and thus it is older women who tend to assert their power over younger women, as Leah's mother-in-law did.[5] As the childless years went by, the pressure from the family became stronger. Yakobo's mother advised him to marry another wife who would could prove that she is capable of bearing children. Yakobo followed his mother's advice and chose Raheli, who had two children with other men before she met Yakobo.

Yakobo sought support from his best man for his decision to desert his wife. The sponsors of the marriage, the best man and matron, are important for a couple long after the actual wedding ceremony is over. According to the constitution of the Northern Diocese, these sponsors of the marriage are the first ones to counsel the young couple in their marriage. Traditionally, they were chosen by the families and were an older, married, and experienced couple. But in contemporary Tanzania, and in the case of Leah and Yakobo, the sponsors were chosen by the couple themselves, although they had to fulfill some requirements set in the constitution, as were previously discussed in connection to Christian marriage

---

4. Bülow, "Power, Prestige," 12.
5. Inhorn, *Infertility and Patriarchy*, 172–74.

in the Northern Diocese. The best man of Yakobo's and Leah's marriage was an influential person in the community, and his strong advice to desert Leah influenced Yakobo to finally encourage Leah to move back to her parent's place.

Yakobo himself stressed the importance of listening to his parents' advice in his sparse narrative. He argued that one should respect elders and follow their advice. Yakobo was proud of his comment that the elders have to be respected. He also maintained that in Chagga culture it is acceptable to marry a second wife if the first one is barren. Yakobo's narrative reveals that he supports the traditions of his patriarchal Chagga community. The social system of Chagga society stresses a man's reproductive role, and it seems that Yakobo felt this strong pressure from his side of the family.[6]

Third-person narrators, both church workers and parishioners, evaluated whether Yakobo made a right decision. Some, as with the pastor in the following account, saw it to be correct to follow the advice of his mother and sponsor.

PASTOR: *When people evaluate his decision they see that he chose correctly. Because it is seen! If he would stay only with this one [. . .]! Today he would die without children and that would be a mistake in the Chagga community, also in Africa. A marriage without children is counted as not a complete marriage.*

This former pastor of the rural parish explained that if Yakobo had stayed only with Leah, he would die without children. He, and others who commented similarly, stressed the African understanding of immortality through procreation and thought it was a wise decision for Yakobo to take another wife. However, not all agreed with his deserting his wife. This group, one older pastor among them, construct their social identity strongly from the *kienyeji* cultural category. They argue that the Chagga traditions have to be followed in the Christian context as well. This is how one young evangelist in the rural parish evaluates the desertion:

EVANGELIST: *Still they saw that this wife is a trustworthy person, and a wife who is well-behaving. And even when they saw this deed [desertion] which was done in such a way. They were amazed and talked about it. They saw that it was not right. And others continue still today to blame him, that husband and they also blame the sponsor because of supporting desertion.*

---

6. Swantz, *Women in Development*, 81–83.

When Leah was deserted, many people in the village considered it as an awful thing and complained. They were especially vocal on the role of the best man in the process of desertion. People in the community consider Leah to be a responsible and trustworthy person who tried her best in the difficult situation. Yakobo's friend did not counsel the husband to stay with his wife as would have been expected of him; instead, he supported advocated desertion. The evangelist and others who do not agree with the desertion of a childless wife stress that a Christian couple should stay committed even though they have no children. From their point of view, there is no need to stress procreation because the Christian belief and hope in immortality through Jesus Christ is enough. Noteworthy in the above account is how the evangelist comments that the procedure of desertion was done in such a way. During the interview he shouted these words and was angry even after a long period of time. The desertion of Leah was, for this evangelist and also for many other people in the rural community, an example of unfair treatment of a childless wife.

These two explanations on Yakobo's decision to desert his wife show how differently the community, including the church, evaluates his decision. In the earlier account the older pastor bases his arguments on Chagga traditions; according to them, the immoral action is to stay childless. Nothing should cut the lineage which must continue. The young evangelist, in the latter account bases his arguments in the Christian setting and found Yakobo's decision to be immoral.

Yakobo lived with Raheli in a distant town, and Raheli gave birth to their first child, a son. Later a second child, a daughter, was born. During the process of desertion, Yakobo was living already with Raheli and their two children. These children were born before Yakobo finally decided to abandon Leah. This seems to indicate that Yakobo wanted to ensure that he could have children with Raheli before chasing Leah away. During that time Leah stayed on the family farm living next door to her parent's-in-law and other members of the patriarchal Chagga family. According to Leah's personal narrative, she did not know about Yakobo having another woman in town before the first child was born. After hearing of a birth of Yakobo's child in town, Leah started to see that her marriage was really in crisis.

The crisis went on and Leah sought help from the pastor of the parish. The pastor, according to Leah's explanation, advised Yakobo to take care of his first wife even if he had married a second one. Leah analyses this crucial stage of their marriage:

LEAH: *They said he should listen to the words of a pastor. Because pastor told him that it is fine if you take another wife as you have done. But you have to know this is your first wife. And the house is hers . . . You cannot tell her to leave. If it is a question of building, build another house aside. Or if it is a room decide that she will get one room and you will stay with the other wife. But the one with a house, the one who has the homestead is the first one! [...] He said if there are children, they should be given to her [the first wife] so that she could raise them. This is how it is: [. . .] give those children to her and she will raise them.*

This account reveals that Leah did not have anything against Yakobo marrying another wife, but only that he should have taken care of her too. Leah agreed that a polygynous marriage would have been a better solution than desertion in her case.

Leah continued her explanation of Chagga tradition in which the first wife always has a higher status. It was not right to make her to move from her home. She used an interesting expression, "The one with the homestead is the first wife," which points to the higher status of being the first wife in her Chagga culture. The higher status of the first wife carries the idea that she should have the right to raise the children born to the second wife. This would bring the first wife the respect, *heshima*, which she should have. *Heshima* is an important word in Swahili, which shows proper behavior in the community. One earns her or his *heshima*, it is not something that can be inherited as property.

Leah was willing to stay in a polygynous marriage but Yakobo decided to separate from her. Yakobo explained that in the contemporary situation it is impossible to live in a polygynous household. His reasons were that it would have been too hard on him to support two wives and that the two women could not cope with each other in one house. Yakobo preferred separation to polygyny. Inhorn found three similar reasons for the preference of divorce over polygyny. The first reason is finance. The second reason is that infertility is a legitimate and socially acceptable excuse for ending a loveless marriage. The third reason to prefer divorce is that most women find the idea of sharing their husband with another wife intolerable.[7]

Leah used the word *mwanamke*, a woman, while talking about Raheli. This word *mwanamke* shows clearly that such a person is not respected as the man's legal wife in the community. A wife, *mke,* is a respected person who has her rights in the community. Raheli's role in the community

---

7. Inhorn, *Infertility and Patriarchy*, 119.

seems to be unclear. Some see her as a second wife, using the word *mke* while referring to her, while others define her role as a cohabiting partner, not an official wife. Yakobo's parents accepted Raheli but the narrative does not reveal how this second relationship was organized within the family. According to the Marriage Act of 1971 a Christian marriage cannot be converted from monogamous to polygynous. Yakobo did not take an official divorce from Leah, so the relationship with Raheli had to be informal.[8]

Leah did not like to discuss this period even after a long time. It had been the hardest time in her life and she did not like to think about these years. She recalls that the family of her husband brought her many problems during that time. Others in the community supported and helped her. Leah recalls that her own family supported her and did not blame her for the difficult situation. Leah's father had already died before this time and so her family was weaker when discussing the problem with Yakobo's family.

Prayer life was important for Leah during these extremely hard years of desertion. She discussed how one cannot know the plans of God, but more important than knowing the exact plan is that a person knows God:

LEAH: *You cannot know how God plans or how he plans your life. But more important is the degree a person knows God. [. . .] And so that what you want to do is to pray. If you pray God and you wait, God will do it.*

AULI: *Yes, you noticed that God really has power?*

LEAH: *Yes, a lot!*

AULI: *Even during the difficulties of life?*

LEAH: *Yes, during those difficulties. [. . .] Even other times even during day time, I use my time for prayer, in the evening again.*

While she told about her prayer life, I wanted to know if she had gone to prayer meetings to be prayed for. Her reply was interesting: "I had done nothing wrong. There was nothing to reconcile, so why would I have gone to a certain healer or even to my local pastor to be healed? I could pray just as well myself." Leah felt that going to ask somebody to pray for her would reveal that she was guilty of something. Because of that, personal prayer was enough for her. She explained earlier how she had gone to see a pastor because of her marital problems, but in this account she explained that she did not seek him for prayer and healing. Relying on God was Leah's way

---

8. Westerlund, "Marriage and Religion," 99.

of coping with her difficult situation. The Christian context was important for Leah during the time of desertion.

Deserter Is Put under Church Discipline

Yakobo lived in town with Raheli and their children. He did not apply for a divorce from Leah but was still officially married to her. His union with Raheli was informal, from the legal and church point of view. He had signed a monogamous contract with Leah, and according to Tanzanian law those marriages signed as monogamous have to stay monogamous. Because of having a relationship outside his marriage, Yakobo was put under church discipline, which meant that he could not participate in the Holy Communion nor take part in church duties.[9]

> PASTOR: *He has not been admitted back to the church because he has not yet given his wife her right. Because we have a procedure this way! If the first wife did not get children but she is alive. Now in order to make the second marriage to be official, according to law he has to dissolve the first marriage. And after the first marriage is dissolved he has to give the first wife those rights that belong to her. He has to build her a house, and to give her a field, a place, where she can do her things, if he has financial possibilities, until God will call her from this life.*

This account gives one explanation of why the separation of Yakobo and Leah was not accepted in the community. A pastor of the rural parish explains that Yakobo refused to give Leah her financial rights according to the Chagga customs after separation. According to the pastor, Chagga customs after separation are such that if the first wife is barren and still alive, the husband should search for an official divorce and also provide the first wife with some financial support and build her a place to live. Leah worked for many years in Yakobo's farm and Yakobo should have paid her or given her a plot of land. This story claims that only after the first wife has received her share is there is a possibility of an official divorce according to the Chagga traditions. The practice of the Northern Diocese differs, however, from the explanation of this pastor. The Northern Diocese does not allow divorce, and so people use the legal process if they wish to get an official divorce and thereby sidestep any compensation or alimony.[10]

---

9. ELCT, Constitution 1986, 66, 71; Smedjebacka, *Lutheran Church*, 218; Matta, "Church Discipline," 29–30.

10. Swai, "Christian Marriage Counselling."

In the above account, the pastor of the rural parish is the same one who agreed in the fourth story that it is good that Yakobo took another wife so as to not remain childless for the rest of his life. From the *kienyeji* setting of this third-person narrator, Yakobo's behavior of adding another wife was not immoral. What was both against the Chagga traditions and improper was the manner in which Yakobo deserted Leah. His behavior did not follow the Chagga traditions, nor did it follow the legal system of the state or the procedure of the Northern Diocese.

Leah's point of view was that Yakobo withdrew himself from the parish when he decided to take a second wife. Leah stressed how she herself was not under church discipline. She points proudly to how she was allowed to join the Holy Communion during and after desertion. This experience convinced Leah that she did not do anything wrong. This sense of behaving correctly was important for her self-esteem during the time of desertion.

Yakobo's situation was different. When separating from his legal wife, he separated himself from the community of his Lutheran parish. To be excommunicated from the parish where he did not live was a smaller shame for him than to spend the rest of his life without children. Excommunication did not affect Yakobo's life much, since he lived away from his home parish in the village.

In one short narrative Yakobo tells a story of how once his son was seriously sick and he carried him to a big stadium where a famous preacher had come to heal people. This preacher prayed for the child and he was healed.[11] Yakobo's story reveals his strong concern for the health of his child, especially in case of his first born son, his heir. Yakobo's narrative further reveals that when in need of healing he went to a charismatic prayer meeting and not to see his own Lutheran pastor. This was easier for him than to go back and repent so as to rejoin his old parish.

During the time of desertion, Leah had a private prayer life and did not attend the charismatic meetings as Yakobo did in his search of healing. There was a marked difference between both the time and the need of healing between these two former spouses. During the time of Leah's desertion, the open-air meetings where Yakobo went were not common in Tanzania. Leah narrates in the account about her prayer life that she did not feel she had any need for reconciliation. Leah's understanding is that when somebody goes to a healer or a prayer meeting, the person has to have done something wrong and needs reconciliation.

---

11. Setel et. al., "Men's Perspectives," 17.

The charismatic meeting in Yakobo's story happened in the 1990s, when such meetings became more common in all of Tanzania. Going to a charismatic meeting was easier for Yakobo because in a big meeting nobody asked him if he was under church discipline. He could come as an anonymous father bringing his child to be healed. Another reason for Yakobo to attend such meetings, which was revealed in third-person narratives, is that Raheli became a born-again Christian later in her life. In the Tanzanian context, a charismatic Christian, one who is born-again, follows strict rules of behavior in his or her life. Raheli, with the other charismatic Christians, started to attend prayer meetings and Bible studies frequently and left her old project of beer brewing. Raheli influenced Yakobo's decision to go to the charismatic meeting with their sick son.

Quite soon after the separation, Leah was chosen to be a church elder. She was given responsibility in the Lutheran parish, which shows her respected status. For her sense of self-esteem, this role and the status it brought her in the community were important. She proudly narrated that she is helping to serve Holy Communion in her present home parish in the town. Eucharist is treated as a sacred thing in the Northern Diocese. Only pastors can administer it, and those lay people who are chosen to collect empty communion cups are chosen carefully. Evangelists, who in the Northern Diocese conduct normal worship services and even funeral services, are not allowed to administer the sacrament, nor can they assist administering it. Eucharist is celebrated only a few times during the year and congregants must prepare themselves to attend. The selection of Leah to help during the Eucharist shows clearly that she, despite her marital problems, was regarded as a faithful parishioner.

Yakobo would not have been chosen to be a church elder in his home parish in the village or in the Lutheran parish in Mwanza town. He had not repented for his sins publicly in his home parish, which could otherwise have given him a letter to the Lutheran parish in Mwanza to introduce him as a full member of the parish.

Yakobo very seldom came to visit his parents in the village and nobody knew when he would come. It was impossible for the pastor to counsel him because of his absence, and he did not seek counseling for himself. In the practice of church discipline, counseling has often been neglected until the time when the one under church discipline requests to be readmitted to the parish.[12] It seems from the third-person narratives that there was no need for the church workers to contact Yakobo during that time when he did not show a desire for repentance.

---

12. Munga, "Understanding and Practice," 38; *Uamsho*, 309.

Raheli and Yakobo lived in Mwanza, a big town where people have migrated from different parts of Tanzania. In this setting it was easier to live in an informal relationship, which would have been more difficult in his home village in Kilimanjaro. Becoming a father, however, gave Yakobo, a respected status even in his home village; now he had fulfilled the Chagga traditional expectations of procreation.

Yakobo lived in tension between his Chagga traditions and his Christian faith.[13] His place in the Chagga community was more important for him than his place in the Lutheran parish. The role of Lutheran home parish was, however, more important for the construction of Leah's positive identity.

Construction of a Positive Identity

Leah returned to her parents' home after being chased away from her husband's homestead. Her father had died earlier and her mother and brother's family accepted her back home. Leah's financial situation in her natal home was very difficult. Her youngest brother and his wife were farming on Leah's parents' land during the time of desertion. They both accepted Leah's return and took good care of her.

Leah's life situation was not easy after separation. Even though she found shelter and support, she knew that her natal family carried the burden of responsibility for her.[14] To take responsibility for feeding an extra mouth is difficult in the hard economic situation of Kilimanjaro. One third-person narrator defined her status thus: "Her honor is that she is at her parent's place." This stresses that Leah is separated and now belongs back with her parents' family, and, importantly, it reveals that Leah belongs somewhere—that she is not a loose woman who goes around trying to find men.

Leah was at her parents' home but she did not want to stay only at home. She was very active in her local parish during this time in her life. The joy of her life was participating in the choir and the women's group in the parish. In spite of the fact that most of the other women were mothers, Leah could join these groups and she found this important for her identity.

LEAH: *Because being in a group and sharing with your friends brings joy to life.*

AULI: *So you got help from the women's group and from the choir?*

---

13. Urio, *Concept of Memory*, 7.
14. Inhorn, *Infertility and Patriarchy*, 122.

LEAH: *Yes. If you stay alone, just on your own, it is not good. But if you join the others, you share ideas together and enjoy the company of others.*

AULI: *And prayers?*

LEAH: *And prayers help.*

AULI: *So during the time of difficulties, [. . .] you joined the other women and they could help you?*

LEAH: *Yes a lot. The women helped me a lot. [. . .] What I see is good, if you have a problem, is that you should not carry it as a big burden all the time. And do not walk around thinking about your problem. Live as all others live. Do not repeat problem, problem, and problem all the time.*

Leah explains that in a difficult life situation such as hers it is important that one does not remain alone but keeps in contact with others. It was important for her to see others and to get new ideas. One of Leah's active coping strategies after her desertion was to be active and join others. She did not use the passive defense mechanisms of withdrawal and isolation, both of which are accepted behavior for a Chagga woman in crisis.

Leah did not want to talk about her problems the whole time but decided to live as normal a life as possible. Her advice to others in a similar situation is to live the same way as others and not to carry the problem with you all the time. Sharing about her experiences was hard for Leah. She explained that it is better not to talk about your problems with others. The reason behind this seems to be that if you keep quiet, the hard memories will be forgotten faster. Leah is a verbally talented person who knows how to express her ideas well, but she was raised in a culture where family secrets should not be discussed with others and she followed that line with her own life experiences as well. Many times during the interviews Leah used the English word "fight" in the middle of Swahili. This word reveals her attitude: she wanted to be strong and to learn to fight in order to find her own place in the community.

Leah decided to look for work in order to improve her financial situation and to find her own place. The pastor of her home parish helped her to find her first job. She was very proud when she explained how she found work, first at a school and later in an institution. When I met her she was working in a third place and proud of having excelled in her work where, due to this, she was always given more and more demanding tasks. Leah wanted to be self-reliant and not bother her relatives with her problems. Her brother and his wife were and are very supportive of Leah, but she did not want to be a burden for them. They have children who are growing and she felt that she would have been a burden had she stayed longer with them.

Another example of this self-reliance is her project of building a house of her own. She explained how she did not have a place of her own where she could live, and because of this, she bought a plot of land and started building a house there. She was happy to explain about her building project:

LEAH: *I have put the roof on. But still I have to add doors, also windows I don't have yet. It will still take time.*

AULI: *When did you start building your house?*

LEAH: *I started such a small thing but it takes a lot of money!*

AULI: *But I see that you are continuing well.*

LEAH: *What could you do? The life of today is such, for the reason . . . as at home . . . my brother has a wife and children, and they grow. If I go there, one sees that I—you become a burden for them, for that family.*

AULI: *And you like to be self-reliant?*

LEAH: *Yes, it is good to be self-reliant, in that way you can be lighter burden to your relatives. [. . .] If you don't (be self-reliant), if you go there you will be a heavy burden for them.*

AULI: *Is it a greater joy if you visit while you are self-reliant?*

LEAH: *Yes, self-reliant. You live in your own place and if someone wishes to visit you, they come to visit.*

In Machame, building a house is understood to be a male responsibility; it does not belong in the realm of normal female behavior. Leah built her house in town because in her home village there is a shortage of land and also, traditionally, it would be harder to build a house in the village. Another reason for not building her house in the village is that Leah has no right of land inheritance, and therefore cannot build in the area of her father's homestead. Remarkable in the above account is how Leah replied to my question about visiting relatives when you have your own place. She replied by pointing out how important it is to have one's own place because then others can visit her. She is not a passive member of her family, but an active one who is visited by her rural relatives. In Kilimanjaro the one who has visitors is respected, and many times people commented on how happy they were when somebody—for example, a pastor—ate at their place. The choice of words shows how hard it was for Leah to be personal. She used second-person singular while actually talking about herself. She wanted to point to things in a more passive way so as not to point to herself as a main character in her life story.

Another indication of Leah's construction of a strong self-esteem is her explanation of the role of foster children in her life:

LEAH: *Here I live with others. At the moment I live with a child of my brother. And I live with the children of my sister. I have children with me at the home all the time. When I was . . . There is another one; I raised him since he was two years old up until the end of secondary. At the moment he is . . . big! He is married! He has a wife.*

AULI: *And with his wife does he come to visit you?*

LEAH: *Totally. He is like my own child.*

Leah conveyed that children have been very important for her during her whole life. The first children came to her when she still lived in Yakobo's place. One child among those foster children is closer to her than others. This boy came to her when he was only two years old. Leah educated him until he finished secondary school. By the time of the interview he was a married man and had two children of his own. Leah's way of expressing the relationship with this young man is interesting. He is as close as her own child would be, but she did not say that he is her child. This young man visits Leah with his family once in a while because they live far away and cannot be a part of her everyday life. She distinguished between the role of social mother, herself, and the biological mother, a relative of hers, for the young man. She has a strong self-esteem as a social mother and stressed in another story how important it is to raise children properly, not only to give birth to them.

Leah did not use much time during the interviews to discuss these children in her life. There seems to be a certain place for them in her life, but she is self-reliant in this way and her identity is not dependent upon these children. Her own identity is to be "Mama Shoo,"[15] an independent working woman. Leah uses the surname of Yakobo and thus carries the name Mama Shoo. Other women of her age are named using the name of their firstborn child. The name Mama Shoo shows that others do not consider the foster child to be Leah's own son; otherwise she would be named using his name. To be called Mama shows that Leah has a respected

---

15. Mama literally means "mother," but is commonly used to mean "Mrs." The name here has been changed.

place in the community through her marriage and that she herself wants to continue to use the family name of Yakobo even after separation. If she had not married she would be called *dada*, which literally means sister.

Leah finds it important for her identity that she has been married. In the Chagga society, unmarried women are stigmatized. She needed a family to move forward and to receive social recognition. Children brought respectability to Leah after the desertion.[16] It is not good for her *heshima* to live on her own, and rumors would start about what type of life she has. Now that she has family, even foster children, living with her, she has a respected status in the urban community.

Such autonomous actions on the part of a woman seem to contrast with the stereotypes about women in Africa. But Leah's actions are not entirely atypical in Machame, where women fight for their own source of income. The Chagga of Kilimanjaro are seen in Tanzania as being well-educated and modern people. This is especially the case in Machame area, where the education of both girls and boys has been important for a long time.[17] Leah herself is not an educated woman, but through her work she has earned a respected status in the community. Again, Leah constructed her identity mainly from traditional male behavior. Working and having a monthly salary have traditionally been connected to male identity in Kilimanjaro. But it seems that Leah, a childless woman, has to work hard to cope with her childlessness, to such extent that she cannot act only as a female but must also take on traditional male responsibilities in order to gain her place in society.

Reunion?

Yakobo and Raheli started having problems in their relationship after many years of living together. Raheli became a born-again Christian and did not want to live with Yakobo any longer. Yakobo moved back to his home village on the mountain while Raheli stayed in town with their children.

During the interview Yakobo explained that it is better for his children to live in town with their mother because they will receive a better education in town. He returned home to take care of his mother after the death of his father. To leave children behind is very unusual for a Chagga man, and it seems to suggest that Raheli dominated him. In patrilineal Chagga society children belong to a husband and are usually raised in his family.

---

16. Haram, *"Women Out of Sight,"* 139.
17. Bülow, "Power, Prestige," 12.

Raheli stays in the house Yakobo built for himself in Mwanza. Yakobo himself explained that Raheli stays in town in order that his children will get a better education. Children are important to Yakobo, and he wants them to have a proper house to live in. Many men who migrate from Kilimanjaro to towns live in rented houses and build a house in their home village. The house in Mwanza shows that Yakobo planned to stay there permanently, that he was not only visiting the town as many other men from Kilimanjaro feel they are doing.[18]

Yakobo currently lives in the house he built for himself, and Leah lives next to his mother's place. The old house is now in bad condition, which indicates that Yakobo has financial difficulties. There are also other signs which show that this man, earlier so financially well-off, is now having financial difficulties. Leah narrated that when she went to visit Yakobo and his mother she brought them some gifts in order to support them. When saying this, she tried to look as neutral as possible but could not hide the joy of showing how well she is managing her life at the moment. Providing financial assistance is a male duty in Chagga culture, but Leah's behavior showed that she is the one who has power.

Yakobo, the firstborn son in his family, has lost his position in the community. His father was the head of lineage, but Yakobo could not hold that position after the death of his father. When discussing this, Yakobo looked sad. As a young man, his future looked promising. He was employed by the government and respected in his childhood community. He followed his parents' advice and now he is back in a house that is falling apart.

Leah's story about a visit from Yakobo reveals his interest of reunion:

LEAH: *He even came to visit me and started to talk. He asked for forgiveness. He came again to ask forgiveness . . . "If we know that we did something wrong . . ." I replied to him that I had forgiven him long ago and did not have a fault. But I said to him if you now are married and you have children, if you leave those children . . . To give birth is not work, more work is to raise children. It would be good you raise those children.*

Leah reminded him of the issue of how much he wanted to have children. Now he has them and he should take care of them. She uses a proverb in the above story, stating that to give birth is not hard work, but it is harder work to raise children. This topic, the importance of raising and educating children, was dealt with many times during the two interviews with Leah. She stressed how there are many people nowadays who give birth to many

---

18. Setel et al., "Men's Perspectives," 11.

children but do not have the strength, either financial or psychological, to take care of them. With her narrative she purports that it is not as important to give birth to children merely to get a status in the community. Her own life reveals that she has earned respect in the community in spite of her infertility. Leah's story asserts her own success and devalues the success of Yakobo. Leah indicated that Yakobo sought to father children but did not take the responsibility for them.

Further, Leah's story seems to point to the idea that Yakobo should have brought his children to be raised by Leah. Leah connected reunion and the children in the same story and this seems to indicate that a reunion could have been possible if she would have been given the children to be raised. As she said herself, to give birth is not as much work as to raise them. In other words, the work Raheli did is not greater than that which Leah could have by raising the children of Yakobo.

Leah continued her evaluation of how she does not have any need for reunion with Yakobo while discussing about her own burial:

LEAH: *It is not enough to find a burial place. It is you yourself . . . in your heart, you have to discuss with your God, and you have to concentrate in order that you would get that eternal inheritance. This body, buried to a place, you can bury it to any place. But what? It is what I fight about, In order to get the inheritance from God, that one that Lord prepared for us. [. . .] This everybody needs to seek strongly.*

AULI: *So the burial place is not that important?*

LEAH: *Yes. Yes, not important. It is more to fight in order to prepare for your later life. After this body is finished, this body, life afterwards, it will be where? It might be that you prepared your life, God will give you reward. You will get this possibility of eternal life. I see that it is much more important than to search big family here this will not last for ever.*

Leah explained that to be buried in the church yard is most important for her. Eternal life is more important than the earthly family life. Eternal inheritance is more important than to have an heir on earth. Leah wants everybody to search for this eternal inheritance and not to concentrate on the earthly life.

The traditional burial place among the Chagga is in the husband's homestead. Leah stressed that this is not important for her. A burial in Yakobo's homestead would be a question of status in the earthly community, but it is not a requirement for eternal life. Eternal life is something greater for Leah, and she wants to fight for a place in heaven. The above account reveals that the *kikristo* cultural category is central for Leah. She relies on Christian immortality through salvation on the cross. Leah does not want to follow the Chagga traditions and wants to show that the ethnic ancestral beliefs are not important for her. She cannot rely on *kienyeji* values because, as a childless, separated wife, she does not have any place or social role in the traditional community.

Leah has other reasons not to accept Yakobo's invitation to return to live as his wife. One of the church workers in the village clarifies how Yakobo is known to have lived a loose life. Leah seemed to be afraid of being infected HIV/AIDS if she would return to Yakobo. Leah would not gain anything, neither status nor financial security, if she would reunite with him. She has both a strong self-esteem and a respected status in the community, to such a degree that she has the power to refuse a reunion. Leah's narrative is her own life story, not only a story of her marriage. Reunion with Yakobo is not her desire, neither in life nor in death. Yakobo would be willing to reunite with Leah, and he seemed to be ready to ask for reconciliation even from his parish.

Tension between Traditional and Modern Values

The narrative of Leah and Yakobo focuses on the stigma of infertility leading to marital separation. The setting of this narrative is the Chagga society, which is in transition. Leah and Yakobo live amidst tension between traditional, Christian, and modern values. This tension brings extra stress to an infertile marriage.

The social changes are happening very fast in Kilimanjaro. The communal ties that used to be the backbone of people's moral behavior have been loosening, especially in the urban situation. Yakobo's migration to town seemed to have influenced the breakdown of his marriage. Urban lifestyle is individualistic; there is less traditional communal control and support for a couple than in the rural village. Some of these separations are only geographical in nature, as was the case with Leah and Yakobo during the early years of their marriage.

The data of this research reveals that most of the references to marital separation were from the rural parish. Only four coded quotations are from the urban setting. One reason for the larger number of references to separation from the rural parish is that in a small village everybody knows about the life of other people. The urban setting is more anonymous and family matters are not known by everybody.

The second frame of reference that influenced the life of this childless couple in Kilimanjaro is *kienyeji*, the traditional way. In the discourse with young people, *kienyeji* is understood to be old-fashioned, something which is against the modern trends. In connection to marital matters, interviewees in Machame stress, however, that it is important to follow the Chagga traditions in order to strengthen the marriages of young people, especially during the time of HIV/AIDS. Hasu comes to a similar conclusion that the fear of HIV/AIDS increases the importance of traditions.[19] People seem to return to search for help from the traditions of their ancestors when they are in trouble.

One of the factors under the *kienyeji* category that adds stress to an infertile couple is family interference. In the rural setting, the family interference seems to be stronger than in the urban setting. The comparison of the model narratives of a committed union and desertion indicate the different influence of urban and rural community. Another factor, indicated in Figure 4, is the patriarchal pressure of the continuation of lineage, which is clearly seen to affect the decisions of a husband to search for a child outside of marriage.

The Christian frame of reference, *kikristo*, is a third contributor to the marital discourse. The village where Yakobo and Leah are from is a dominantly Lutheran community. The teachings of the local parish influence the marital life of the parishioners. The workers of the local parish were able to define the problems of the Christian marriages in their parish. Many pointed to the ineffectiveness of church discipline and lack of counseling while discussing the case of Leah and Yakobo.

The church workers, especially pastors and evangelists, take an active role in community matters in Kilimanjaro. These church workers are not only responsible for the spiritual work of the parish, but they are responsible for many practical things in the community. For example, they are responsible for marriage counseling and seeking restoration in various other crisis situations. Church discipline is one of the tools used to control the life of parishioners. However, many parishioners and church workers criticize the practice of church discipline. The critics consider it an outdated practice that does not help the situation in contemporary Kilimanjaro.

The role of the sponsors of a marriage was found to be problematic in the narrative of desertion. It seems that unclear social identification brings problems to the system of marriage sponsors. Many times these sponsors are selected to fit the requirements of the Chagga community, not in order to serve as suitable Christian counselors. Many of these sponsors who

---

19. Hasu, *Desire and Death*, 240–43.

try to counsel couples live in the same tension between traditional and Christian expectations as the newly married themselves.

The third-person narratives of church workers did not always follow the *kikristo* cultural category. The findings of this chapter reveal that one of the church workers identified himself more strongly with the Chagga traditions than other interviewees among the church workers. One young evangelist constructed his social identity mainly from the Christian setting. The church is in the middle of this tension between traditional and modern values, and it has not defined its stance towards either the tradition or the contemporary situation.

One of the issues that bring hot debates in contemporary Kilimanjaro is divorce. The Lutheran church in Tanzania teaches strongly against divorce despite the fact that many of its parishioners are actually living separated from their spouses or are seeking official divorce. To get approval for an official divorce in the church, the case must start at the parish level and then go to the district level. Only later it is taken to the diocese to be discussed. Many who wish to be divorced do so by going through the court and do not get approval through the church.[20] The advice offered by the church is usually that the couple should tolerate the situation and stay together.

The sample of this study does not reveal the whole situation of the childless divorcée in Kilimanjaro because the interviewed divorcées were all active parishioners. The possibility of prostitution was not even mentioned in my data. The social system of the Chagga differs from that of the Haya of Bukoba where many childless divorcées seem to end up as prostitutes. This does not seem to be common among the Chagga.[21]

The findings of the model narrative of desertion reveal that Leah was very much on her own, suffering under the pressure from Yakobo's family and from the life situation when Yakobo had migrated to town. She learned to cope with her infertility stigma and to build a new, independent identity. The desertion of Leah, socially, sexually, and financially, created a strong middle-aged woman. Leah gained a positive identity and learned to cope with her infertility. She does not need children as a tool to have a place in a community. She has earned a respected place within the community through her own identity and achievement. It seems, however, that in order to achieve respected status, Leah had to sacrifice much of her female identity and traditional female behavior. She constructed her independent identity from traditional male characteristics. It seems that a

20. Swai, "Christian Marriage Counselling."
21. Swantz, *Women in Development*, 83; Larsson, *Conversion*, 96–99, 120, 139.

childless woman has to be as strong as a man in order to be accepted in the Chagga society. Leah earned her place within the community by showing that she is capable of taking on the traditional male responsibilities. Leah is not under patriarchal control because she can take care of herself in all aspects of life, including planning her own funeral. Such autonomous actions as seen in Leah's behavior contrast with the stereotypes about African women. Leah's actions are not entirely atypical in Machame, where many women are strong and at least partly self-reliant.

The traditional role identity of a Chagga wife is to be a peasant wife who does the farming on her husband's farm. This was Leah's role before her separation from Yakobo. After the separation, Leah did not have a farm or cows any longer and she had to learn to become a wage laborer in a different field. She moved to town because of her work and she established an independent role there. When living in a traditional homestead, Leah's social identity was *kienyeji*, and she fulfilled the traditional requirements of a good wife. After the separation she could no longer depend on *kienyeji*, but instead she constructed a new role identity as a working woman. Leah's new identity belongs to cultural categories *kisasa* and *kikristo*. In part she still follows *kienyeji*, especially in her need to have children to safeguard her respected status in the community.

With Yakobo the main problem seems to be his relationship to his community. In the African context, the collective self is important and one's life has meaning only when it supports and strengthens the collective self. True death is the exclusion of the individual from the community.[22] Yakobo followed the advice of Chagga traditions in his life, but he did not fulfill these regulations, either. This seems to be his problem. He constructed his social identity partly from the *kienyeji* cultural category and partly from hte *kisasa* frame of reference, but he embraced neither one of these value groups. However, as a result when he separated for the second time, he was left alone to deal with his problems. Yakobo's interest in the charismatic meetings reveals, however, that he has a need to cope with his past. Also, the quest for reunion reveals Yakobo's need for reconciliation with Leah and with his Lutheran home parish.

The narrative of desertion explains how a Chagga man has difficulties in building a male identity in a changing Tanzania. At the end of his personal story, the situation of Yakobo is not good. He has lost almost everything in his life: his legal wife, his children, his long time companion, his wealth, and his position in society and in the church. He is still under church discipline, and if he is not reunited to the parish before his

---

22. Masamba ma Mpolo, "Spirituality and Counselling," 19.

death he will be denied a church burial. The parish seems to support Leah's decision not to reunite and this makes Yakobo's situation even worse. He does not get support for his plans to reunite, even from the church, which usually instructs to reconcile the marriage and advises the wife to tolerate and to forgive.

Leah and Yakobo used individual but not joint coping strategies, as in the model narrative in chapter 2. Leah's selection of coping strategies shows the importance of church community in her life. Yakobo's selection of coping strategies shows what a traditionally oriented Chagga man he is. His only coping strategy, which cannot be grouped under *kienyeji*, is his interest in charismatic Christianity. Charismatic Christianity shows an interest in modern influences but does not contradict the traditional ways either.

The model narrative of desertion demonstrates how infertility is a problem for both a wife and a husband in Kilimanjaro. Infertility affects Chagga couples in such a way that in most of the cases the result is either marital separation or polygyny, which will be discussed in the following chapter.

4

Two Narratives of Polygyny

Formal Polygyny as a Traditional Coping Strategy

THIS CHAPTER FOCUSES ON the marital crisis of infertility leading to polygynous marriage. Polygyny is a traditional marital arrangement among the Chagga, but is not officially accepted by the Northern Diocese. The life story of Nehemiah and his two wives illustrates a socially accepted formal polygynous marriage in a Chagga context.

Nehemiah and Sarah were young people in a village community. Nehemiah was farming the plot of land given to him by his father. Sarah was an attractive and hard-working young girl from a neighboring village. Nehemiah and Sarah both come from Lutheran families and their church wedding was a big event in the area.

Two years after their marriage Sarah was not yet pregnant. The young couple did not know what to do with the problem. Family members advised them to search for a reason for their infertility. Sarah and Nehemiah went around for two years searching for the reason. They went to a local medical doctor, as well as to a traditional healer, and also conducted sacrifices to the ancestors. The reason for not conceiving was not found through their tireless investigation, therefore no cure was found. The demand to find a reason brought some confrontations between Nehemiah and Sarah. They were both getting tired of using their time and money in search of a reason for their infertility.

Finally Nehemiah and Sarah met someone who worked for Kilimanjaro Christian Medical Centre (KCMC), the big university hospital in Moshi. This third-person narrator, an evangelist of the rural parish, explained the meeting with this person:

EVANGELIST: *He went even to the traditional healers because his wife and he himself were so desperate. Fortunately, when they came, there is one person, who works in the KCMC. We told him, you should go to see that one of KCMC. He went and she was examined and was told that your wife has distension in her fallopian tubes. And because of that it is not easy to get a child any longer. And because of that we advise you . . . That distension has to be operated and her whole uterus has to be taken away. But he said that I love that wife so much that I ask you help me to take care of her, she has to be operated.*

In these investigations it was found out that Sarah had problems in her fallopian tubes. This problem was severe and Sarah had to be operated on. This third-person narrator, in telling their story, explained how the doctors of KCMC took Sarah's uterus out. Sarah had to learn to cope with the reality that her infertility was permanent. The narrative of the operation seems to stress the permanent nature of Sarah's infertility and the impossibility for a woman to give birth without a uterus.

The explanation is not meant to give clear medical diagnosis of Sarah's infertility problem. The most important message in the above account is that Nehemiah and Sarah found the reason for their infertility problem. The evangelist was delighted that the reason was found through official medicine and not through a traditional healer or through sacrifices. The official stand of the Northern Diocese is that traditional healers and sacrifices belong only to the Chagga traditional religion and should not be consulted by its parishioners. Many parishioners consult the traditional healers and conduct sacrifices to ancestors, but they do it secretly because it is not allowed. In this case, we clearly see the tension between the *kikristo* and *kienyeji* frames of reference.

The evangelist explained that Sarah's infertility is permanent and seemed to stress that in this case polygyny became an accepted situation. The evangelist manifested a contradiction here: he seemed to accept the polygynous marriage of Nehemiah while knowing that the Northern Diocese does not officially accept it. This is not the same evangelist as in the case of Leah and Yakobo, who based his arguments in the *kikristo* category. The evangelist here seemed to use more of the *kienyeji* category to approve the decision of Nehemiah to find another wife.

After the operation Sarah noticed that Nehemiah was becoming depressed, and his love for her decreased. Nehemiah did not blame Sarah for her physical problem because the doctors had explained that the reason for Sarah's infertility had been an untreated infection when she was a child. This third-person narrator, a female pastor in the rural parish, explained the situation after Sarah's operation:

PASTOR: *When the first wife saw that love was decreasing she gave the husband a permission to marry another wife so that she would not be beaten and that food would come home. And then that man went and married that concubine. He brought her home and they were now two women in the house.*

This account reveals that Sarah wanted to save her marriage and secure her own financial situation. She was also afraid that Nehemiah, in his depression due to not having a child, would become violent toward her. Sarah gave Nehemiah permission to marry a second wife in order to secure her own place in the family. Nehemiah took a second wife, Neema ("Grace"), who gave birth to his first child, and later on, to other children. Neema became a solution for Sarah and Nehemiah's marriage.

The female pastor of the rural parish who gave the above narrative explained from Sarah's point of view. She seemed to understand Sarah's concern for the difficulties in the relationship with Nehemiah, as well as her concern for the financial difficulties that might affect her in a childless marriage. Generally, this female pastor seemed to propose that formal polygyny is a good solution to a childless marriage. Her choice of words in explaining Nehemiah's second marriage is interesting. In referring to the second wife she did not use the normal word *mke*, a wife, but instead she used a negative word, *hawara*, which can be translated to mean concubine, lover, or mistress. Even though she stressed polygyny as a traditional coping strategy, her word choice reveals that she does not completely accept the situation of having a second wife. She seemed to support Sarah, but not particularly Neema, whom she calls a concubine. Nehemiah's family calls her "a wife" and accepts her fully. Following the Chagga traditions, the role of Neema in the polygynous family is always to be the second wife. Sarah is the first wife who takes responsibility of the household.

The pastor of the parish visited Nehemiah and his two wives. She told about her visit to the polygynous household and described the family situation from the parish point of view:

PASTOR: *And the first wife said, pastor, I gave him permission. If you tell my husband to desert the young one (the second wife) . . . [. . .] He asked me, where I should put the other wife? I love them both and I caused her to be crushed. And the second wife said, you should build me a house and I would leave. But the man did not have the money to build a house. And she knew that the husband likes her a lot, also. Because of that it was really difficult. That man . . . I baptized children and the husband stayed as before.*

During her pastoral visit, the pastor told Nehemiah that he should leave one of his wives. At that point Sarah commented that she is the one who gave Nehemiah permission to marry another wife. If Nehemiah should desert Neema, what would her situation be? Nehemiah explained to the pastor how he loved both of his wives, how could he choose between them? As a reason for the difficulty in choosing one, Nehemiah commented that he is the one who crushed Neema, meaning he is the one who took her virginity and whose child she bore. Neema, the shy young wife, raised her voice during the pastor's visit and commented that she would be ready to go if this would make the situation better.

The final decision of the family was that the pastor would baptize the children and the polygynous union would continue as it was. This third-person narrative illustrates polygyny as a pastoral problem. The pastor decided to baptize the two children to whom Neema had given birth but the spouses were left under church discipline. The above account does not reveal if all of the spouses were under church discipline, or if only Nehemiah and Neema were under it, as would be the normal practice of the Northern Diocese. It is interesting to note in this account what strong characters both of the women are. Nehemiah is not the only one who replied to the pastor during her visit, but both of the wives took the responsibility for the marital situation.

The harmonious marital situation is further explained in the following account, which was told by an evangelist of the rural parish:

EVANGELIST: *But in their relationship there was no problem. Even the children do not have problems, they respect them and the children were also respected.*

AULI: *So even the children saw that it was a good plan?*

EVANGELIST: *Yes, and even the church did receive them back to the parish and then . . .*

AULI: *They were officially members of the parish?*

EVANGELIST: *Yes.*

AULI: *These people that you explained to me, how was it, was it so that the first wife lived on her own or did she get some children of the other wife so that she would take care of them?*

EVANGELIST: *It was so that the children of the second wife saw the first wife to be just as their own mother.*

AULI: *So the first wife was equally a mother?*

EVANGELIST: *So even to live, they could stay wherever.*

The evangelist explained the relationship of Nehemiah's two wives and stressed how well they cope with each other. His story also reveals that the children have an official status in the family. After explaining these relationships in the family, he commented on how the church received them back into the parish. This comment came so fast in the middle of an explanation about the relationships that I had to ask again if they were now officially members of the parish. I did not clarify more about the procedure of taking them back, nor did I ask more closely who were received back into the parish. After that short question I returned to the theme that starts the above account. I wanted to know if there was an equal relationship between Nehemiah's two wives and whether they were also equal in terms of motherhood. The interpretation of the evangelist was that the children also treated both of the wives as their mothers. Neema was their biological mother, Sarah a highly respected social mother. Both wives raised the children Neema bore to Nehemiah, but Sarah was given the respected status of the first wife.

Sarah herself could not explain what her life is like as an infertile Chagga woman during her informal interview. The only explanation she had was that it is God's decree that she does not have her own children. While commenting on this, she looked a bit sad and searched for help from Neema and Nehemiah who were both present. Nehemiah and Neema kept quiet but nodded their heads as agreeing to the fact that it was God's plan that Sarah did not give birth.

I wanted to interview Sarah officially another time to ask more what she meant by "decree of God" and also to get her personal life story. During my visit to the rural parish, I heard that old Sarah had passed away. An evangelist of the rural parish narrates the funeral service for Sarah:

EVANGELIST: *Even the one who died a month ago, the children gave her a big respect, if it was a coffin for carrying her corpse to burial. They carried . . . and also that second wife she gave respect to her.*

AULI: *So it was not seen that she did not have children?*

EVANGELIST: *No, it was not easy to see . . .*

Sarah was respected as the first wife and as a social mother of Nehemiah's children even at the time of her death. The funeral service was done in the church quite close to the homestead. After the funeral service Sarah was buried in Nehemiah's homestead by the pastor of the parish. The above explanation does not indicate if there had been any signs or rituals to indicate that the deceased one died without biological children. Many interviewees recalled Chagga traditions that require special rituals to be performed during the burial of a childless wife. In Sarah's case, it seems that these rituals were not needed, or else the narrator either did not know about them or did not want to tell me about them.

Nehemiah and his two wives is a model narrative of older people, and of the three spouses only two are still alive today. Among the Chagga Christians, the practice of formal polygyny is becoming less common. Formal polygyny does not seem to be such a great challenge to the Christian marriage any longer, although informal polygyny remains. Informal polygyny will be discussed more closely in the following section.

Informal Polygyny Supports Male Status

This story about Filipo and his two wives is a model narrative of informal polygyny in contemporary Kilimanjaro. The focus is the lack of a son which leads Filipo to having another wife. As the narrative tells, Filipo has daughters with Blandina, but she is considered to be childless because there are no sons. Traditionally only male children were counted, and giving birth to only female children was included among the traditional reasons for divorce.[1] With informal polygyny I refer to the situation in which the husband has one wife in a village and another wife in a town.

Filipo was a businessman involved in petty trading in Moshi town. Filipo married Blandina from another village in Machame. They live together in the home village and Filipo commuted to Moshi town to do his business. Their first child, Juliana, was born only a few months after both families agreed to a customary marriage. The bride wealth transactions started normally after these agreements.[2] The marriage of Filipo and Blandina was later blessed in their local Lutheran church during the same service where their firstborn Juliana was baptized. The young couple seemed happy and both sides of the family agreed with the marriage arrangements.

Years pass and Mama Juliana[3] gave birth to three other children, all of them girls. Filipo stressed how, in order to meet the needs of a big family, he should have a room to stay in town and not commute every day. The trip back to the village is difficult and expensive. After some time, Mama Juliana came to the conclusion that there had to be another wife in town because Filipo did not bring as much money home any longer, nor did

1. Marealle, *Maisha ya Mchagga*, 48–49.
2. Hasu, *Desire and Death*, 89–96, 253–66.
3. After the birth of her first child she is no longer called Blandina, but Mama Juliana (a pseudonym).

he visit home every weekend as he used to. Also, while visiting he would become quite cranky and violent against Mama Juliana.

The marital situation became worse and Mama Juliana returned to her parents' place. She stayed there for a few months but came to feel that it was not her place any longer; it is now the home of her brother. When leaving she had to leave her children with her husband's family and this was also very hard for her.

Now she feels that it is better to live with her children close to her in-laws even though she does not have a good relationship with them. In order to explain this lack of trust with her in-laws, Mama Juliana narrated a story of how she was sick and had to be taken into Machame hospital for two days. Upon returning home she noticed that the children had been on their own for the whole time. The mother-in-law and other relatives had not come to take care of her young children.

Mama Juliana was very worried when she told the above story in her informal interview, and stressed that this is not how a Chagga family should look after its members. It seems that Filipo's parents do not know how to handle the marital situation of their son and, partly because of this, do not have regular contacts with their daughter-in-law, who lives next door. Another reason for the lack of communication between Mama Juliana and her in-laws is the fact that Filipo is away so much. During the years he lived in the village with Mama Juliana and their children, there were natural contacts with his parents every day.

Even though the situation in the village is not easy, divorce is not a choice for Mama Juliana. Informal polygyny is more accepted in the community than divorce. This situation gives her some independence and she does have a place where she can live. If she were divorced, she would leave her children behind and her financial situation would be much worse. Now what makes her life hard is that she lives close to her in-laws without having a good relationship with them.

Mama Juliana has reasons to stay in her marriage other than to live with her daughters. Mama Juliana discusses her burial plans. She does not want to be buried in a way that would reveal to everybody that her marriage was not working. She wants to keep the facade in order to be buried properly in her husband's homestead. This proper burial will also grant her daughters official status in the family. For Mama Juliana, the social acceptance of the community is important. She seemed to stress that the life here on earth is not the only one.

Women face gender oppression beyond the grave. They have to think of their status even while planning their burial. Burial is more than a question of individual choice; it indicates the deceased's status in the community. Mama Juliana's comment also shows the importance of the ancestors as a part of the community. She feels that if she were officially divorced and not properly buried in her husband's banana grove, this would decrease her chance of becoming a "living dead" in the family of her husband. Those who are already dead but are still remembered in the community are called living dead.[4]

Filipo's *mke mdogo* is named Upendo in this model narrative, and her name means love. Literally, *Mke mdogo* means "second wife" or "younger wife," but its use in everyday language comes closer to the meaning of a concubine. It is most common that a concubine is in town, but there are also cases where both women are in the same village, although not in the same homestead as is the case in traditional polygyny.[5]

Upendo asserted that she has a good relationship with Blandina in her short personal account:

UPENDO: *If I meet his wife, I see her as a normal person. There is no quarrel . . .*

Upendo explained that she has good relationship with Filipo's formal wife. However, Blandina did not agree with Upendo's interpretation, and discussed Filipo's life in town critically.

Upendo openly admitted during her interview that her six children are born from different fathers. Now she lives in a suburb of Moshi with Filipo, who is the father of her two youngest children, both sons. She explained that she wanted to have many children because she loves them. Others in the suburban community see Upendo as somebody who has children in order to guarantee financial security in her own life. The third-person narrators claimed that she did not actually want to have more children, but has them in order to keep Filipo's support.[6] One neighbor woman interpreted the economic value of children for Upendo this way:

MRS: *She does not have the financial possibilities for self-reliance. She is not a woman who likes to work with her hands. She likes to sell small things like onions . . . [. . .] She has quite many children and she has children with different men. The reason of having children is to meet her financial needs. So that she could get her basic needs.*

---

4. See Mbiti, *African Religions*, 25.
5. Kanyongo-Male and Onyango, *Sociology*, 106; Waruta, "Marriage and Family," 108; Schoepf, "Inscribing the Body Politic," 111.
6. Hasu, *Desire and Death*, 322–29.

The neighboring woman used quite strong words to define Upendo. She dod not say it openly, but her idea seems to be that Upendo is a loose woman who has men in order to meet her financial needs. Her interpretation was that Upendo searches for children in order to bind men to stay longer with her. She did not even regard Upendo as living in a marital situation with Filipo.

Filipo was put under church discipline when the pastor of the rural parish learned about Upendo. The female pastor of the urban parish discussed Filipo's situation and the role of his first child born with Upendo in the following account.

> PASTOR: *From the side of the church he will be put under church discipline. He has to be put under discipline because he acted against his marriage. In the society and in the family that the child who was born outside of marriage, if the father admits that is his! The customs and traditions will give that child all rights. That child, he has no fault. And father says that is mine because I did not get a child so I got him, he is my child. He has the inheritance rights. [. . .] And in that family father went to search a male!*

This account reveals again the tension between church discipline and the Chagga traditions. Filipo is put under church discipline because of having a child outside his marriage. However, even the pastor who has seen him living with Upendo in the urban area agreed that the child will get all his rights, including inheritance.

Mama Juliana is not under church discipline, and she was chosen to be a parish elder even after the polygynous situation was known in the community. Now Mama Juliana raises her children mainly on her own in the rural village, and Filipo usually visits them only once a month. Upendo and Filipo live together as a family in the urban setting in an informal relationship.

Both narratives in this chapter reveal that church workers have difficulties in handling polygynous marriages. Both polygynous men, Nehemiah and Filipo, were put under church discipline. The following section compares the findings of the two narratives of polygyny to the findings of the narrative on desertion.

Separation or Adding Another Wife?

Among the Chagga polygyny is a traditionally accepted solution for an infertile marriage. Separation, however, seems to be a more common practice than traditional polygyny in contemporary Kilimanjaro. This section evaluates the findings of the model narratives on desertion and polygyny.

A single reading through the model narratives of desertion and informal polygyny gives the impression that the stories are quite similar. The difference between them is in the different decisions of the two men from the same village. Yakobo deserted his wife Leah and chose to live only with Raheli in town. Filipo continued his marriage with Mama Juliana and visits her regularly although not frequently. Filipo supports Mama Juliana and their daughters financially. From the narrative it seems that Filipo and Mama Juliana also continues to have a sexual relationship, which was not the case with Leah and Yakobo after the desertion. Filipo's polygynous situation is unclear in the eyes of the community, but it is clearly a polygynous situation and not a separation, as is the case of Leah and Yakobo.

The situation of both first wives, Leah and Mama Juliana, is also quite different. Mama Juliana is a mother and she has to think about her daughters' lives. She could not, even if she tried, leave the difficult marital situation and start an independent life on her own as Leah did. The desire for a place of funeral is different between these two active parishioners. Leah asserted in her narrative that the only place to be buried is in the church yard, while Mama Juliana stressed that she wants to be buried properly in the homestead of her husband. Leah constructed her social identity strongly from the *kikristo* category. Mama Juliana expressed her wish to follow the Chagga traditions. These two model narratives further reveal that a separated wife has the freedom to live an independent life in contemporary society, but a wife who lives in informal polygyny, especially one who lives in the homestead of her husband's family, has to tolerate the patriarchal family and society at large.

The two narratives of polygyny discussed in this chapter are quite different. In Nehemiah and Sarah's case, the first wife agreed for her husband to marry another wife. In the second narrative, Filipo did not even inform Mama Juliana that he had taken another wife in town. Mama Juliana suspected this for some time and later heard about Upendo from her neighbors. In the case of formal polygyny, the relatives of both Nehemiah and Sarah agreed upon it and saw it as a good decision in order to save a childless marriage. Table 6 compares the differences in the narratives of Nehemiah's and Filipo's polygynous marriages.

Table 6: The Differences between Two Polygynous Marriages

Nehemiah	Filipo
Reason for Sarah's infertility is known	Mama Juliana gives birth only to girls
Permission from Sarah to take another wife	No permission from Mama Juliana to take another wife
Community accepts polygyny	Community seems to hesitate with informal polygyny
Church community understands decision to marry another wife	Church community condemns Filipo's decision to have a concubine
Nehemiah was under church discipline	Filipo is under church discipline
Rural setting and all three spouses live together	Rural (Mama Juliana) and urban (Upendo) settings
Two nowadays old people, first wife has died	A middle aged couple and a young concubine.
Sarah, Neema and Nehemiah are from the same village	Mama Juliana is from another village in Machame and Upendo is from Marangu, in East Kilimanjaro.

Formal polygyny seems to provide more respect to all those involved. Informal polygyny generally mistreats all persons involved. Often the husband is pressured to desert his wife or to beget children outside of the marriage. The role of the infertile wife is not easy; her status is low. The role of the second wife is very insecure. If the husband is only searching for a child from this type of a relationship, the second woman might lose her child to the household of the husband and his barren wife. The other possibility is that the child is taken care of by her mother but she will never have the official status and security of a married wife.

The effects of informal polygyny on the first marriage are many. The economic effects are serious: in many cases, the husband takes most of the wealth from the first family and spends it on the second family. Children born in the first marriage often feel that their father has left them and does not care for them any more.

The psychological effects on the first wife generally make her life more difficult. She has to take the responsibility for the whole family but she is not given the means to do it. At the same time, she often feels deserted. When a husband has an affair outside marriage or has an informal wife, this ruins the interdependent relationship in the Christian marriage. In addition to the other effects on the first wife, there is a fear of contracting HIV/AIDS. Extramarital relationships and informal polygyny tend to increase the spread of STDs, in comparison to traditional polygyny in which a second wife is added to the same homestead.[7]

The risk of STDs increases when there are more sexual partners, as is the case with a *mke mdogo* who has children from various men. Even if the husband does not have sex with more women than his formal and informal wife, when entering his *mke mdogo's* "sexual web" the possibility of getting HIV/AIDS becomes much higher in comparison to the situation of three committed spouses as in the case of traditional polygynous marriage. Thus, an infertile wife or a wife who has only girls is in greater danger of being infected from the broad "sexual web" of her husband.

One reason for informal polygyny seems to be the desire for children. In traditional Chagga society it was important to have a wife or wives in order to produce as many children as possible, thereby ensuring the continuation of the lineage.[8] While the desire for children remains important in the contemporary society, there is an increasing use of some family planning techniques.

The gender of a child remains important, not only the number of children, as is seen from Filipo's desire for a son. Male children are valued in patrilineal Chagga society because, while female children will be married to another family, males are those who traditionally stay to take care of their parents. In the past, having many wives was a sign of wealth and status in the traditional Chagga community. Nowadays, to have an informal wife seems to give a modern man a higher status in the community. Only a rich person can financially support two or more women. Polygyny apparently remains connected to the power and social status of Chagga men. The role of women is not so central in polygyny, especially the role of the second wife, which is often undefined.

Second Wife—an Incubator or a Spouse?

The discussion about polygyny as a strategy to cope with childlessness concentrates mainly on the husband and his first wife. The role of a second wife is not often discussed in the narratives on childlessness in Kilimanjaro. The

---

7. Ngavatula, "Concept of Adumile," 31–40.
8. Njuu, "Traditional Marriage," 18; Omari, "Fertility Rates," 259.

question is whether the second wife is a true spouse with her own rights or just an instrument to produce children to save a childless marriage. Table 7 compares the life stories of the three second wives and evaluates their role in the family. The titles I have given to these women are an interpretation of their status in the family and in the larger community.

Table 7: Comparison of the Lives of Three Second Wives

Neema, Formal Second Wife	Raheli, Cohabiting Partner	Upendo, Concubine
Rural	Urban	Urban
Children only with Nehemiah	Children with many men	Children with many men
Was married because of the advice of the first wife	Relationship started without the knowledge of the first wife	Relationship started without the knowledge of the first wife
Lives in the same homestead with Nehemiah and Sarah, has her own small hut	Lives in a house built by Yakobo	Lives in a rented house, Filipo pays the rent
Formal second wife	Separation of Leah and Yakobo was not official making Raheli's situation unclear	No formal agreement on polygyny; her status is as concubine
Accepted by parents-in-law	Accepted by parents-in-law	No clear relationship with parents-in-law
Lutheran, not under church discipline	Previous denomination not known, recently born-again, Charismatic Christian	Lutheran, under church discipline
Polygynous marriage continued until recently, children are adults, the two old spouses have two grandchildren to live with them in the village, and Sarah died during the field research	Now separated from Yakobo, lives with her children in town	Lives with Filipo and all her children in town, claims to have good relationship with Mama Juliana

There is also a practical reason for informal polygyny among those Chagga men who have migrated to towns in search of work. These men need somebody to take care of their domestic tasks in town. In an urban situation without running water or a washing machine, the normal domestic tasks are a time-consuming burden for men living on their own. It is easier and cheaper to have an *mke mdogo* than to hire a maid.

The purpose of a second wife seems to be to produce children. The relationship between a husband and his wives is not interdependent in a traditional Chagga marriage. The man is clearly the head of the family in a polygynous household. The role of a cohabiting partner is slightly more independent. Raheli was not only an incubator to give birth to Yakobo's children, but also Yakobo's only partner during the time they lived together. Her role can not truly be described only as an incubator of babies. Upendo, among our examples of second wives, is the closest to being an incubator. She was clearly chosen to give birth to a son, but she is also a spouse with whom Filipo lives. During the interviews, many third-person narrators told about such women who give birth to a child who is then raised in the infertile family. I did not personally encounter this type of childless family or any such woman whose role was only as an incubator. Most probably there are such cases, but I doubt if they are as common as the interviewees seemed to purport. Polygyny, which was an accepted practice in the traditional Chagga society, remains one of the challenges to Christian marriage as will be more closely discussed in the following section.

Polygyny as a Pastoral Problem in the Northern Diocese

Already in the 1930s polygyny was understood to be a pastoral problem among the Chaggas. Hasu maintains, "From the male perspective polygyny was one of the arenas on which local culture and social hierarchy confronted Christianity and on which that hierarchy was contested."[9] Since the time of the first missionaries, church discipline was used in cases of polygyny.[10] Polygyny is still today a pastoral problem and some parishioners are under church discipline because of it.

Polygyny has been a widely discussed topic in African theology since the 1960s.[11] There are different policies concerning polygyny in various dioceses of the ELCT. In the Arusha Diocese, which has many polygynous marriages, a man with many wives can be baptized in the Lutheran church

---

9. Hasu, *Desire and Death*, 159.
10. Ibid., 164–65.
11. Mbiti, *Love and Marriage*, 81–82.

but cannot add another wife after that. The members in Arusha Diocese are predominantly from either an Arusha or Maasai ethnic background, both of which are strongly polygynous cultures.

In the Northern Diocese, only monogamous marriages are allowed, and the number of formally polygynous marriages among Lutheran Christians is quite small. The constitution of the Northern Diocese discusses polygyny both in connection with those who are permitted to have a church wedding and in connection to divorce. Marriage is not officiated for those who are under church discipline, which includes all known polygynists.[12]

According to the Northern Diocese constitution, it is a sin to break a marriage. This is further defined as a married "Christian" husband taking another wife, or a married "Christian" wife being taken by another husband.[13] Noteworthy is the active role given to men. In those cases where the one breaking the marriage is a woman, her deed is described in a passive form; she is taken by another man. It seems that there is strong influence from the Chagga culture in the constitution of the Northern Diocese. In the Chagga understanding a man is the one who marries, and this understanding has influenced the wording of the constitution.

There was active discussion about polygyny among parishioners in Kilimanjaro. In the coding category "polygyny," all references to polygyny are included and no differentiation is made between formal and informal polygyny. The interviewees from the rural community referred to polygyny three times more often than those from the urban parish. These findings from the results of coding categories seem to confirm that polygyny is a traditional strategy used to cope with childlessness, and referring to it is more natural in the rural than in the urban community.

Childless persons themselves and the workers of both these parishes commented regularly about polygyny as a strategy to cope with childlessness. In references to the coding category, polygyny was used rather infrequently with the parishioners, even though some of the parishioners commented more often on polygyny during informal discussions. It seems that those who are concerned about the effects of childlessness in their own marriage and those working in counseling in local parishes did consider polygyny more often than the normal parishioners or the other parish workers. It must be noted, however, than the sample of such other parish workers is very small. Only two people were interviewed who worked in the parishes but were not pastors or evangelists.

12. ELCT, Constitution 1986, 70.
13. Ibid., 73.

Male informants referred to polygyny more often than did female interviewees. The attitude of males toward polygyny was also more positive than the attitude of female interviewees. This gender difference in references to polygyny becomes more significant when we consider that the total number of males in the sample is much less than the number of females, as was discussed in chapter 1. Some women seemed to consider polygyny as a good coping strategy. Other women did not comment on polygyny, or they thought it was suited only to traditional society, not to contemporary Chagga community.

Pastors of both study parishes stressed that the need to have a child is one reason to delay the sealing of a marriage in a church. To have children is a must, and the church does not offer divorce as an option. It is easier to wait until the first child is born. Setel et al. collected the data of their research among young men in Moshi town and found out that many men preferred a wife who was proven to be fertile.[14]

The traditional marriage arrangements were an affair of the whole community. The families were both involved and responsible for preparing the young couple for marriage. We can see the importance of the community in Nehemiah's case and also, negatively, in the lack of support from family in Filipo's case.

Bride wealth often acts as the uniting element between the two families. These payments secure the situation of the marriage. Some people commented during the field research that bride wealth is an old-fashioned practice and is no longer used. From my observations, it seems that this is not completely true. There seems to be some bride wealth transactions in almost all of the more recognized unions. The amount of bride wealth differs depending on whether it is an official church marriage or a customary marriage.

Many female theologians in Africa criticize polygyny as being a way to exploit women.[15] The findings of the model narrative on formal polygyny suggest, however, that there are some good aspects of traditional polygyny, even for the women. The way parishes deal with polygyny often brings problems to Christian couples. Church discipline does not relieve the pressure of the traditional Chagga community towards procreation.

The contemporary Chagga community is in transition. Urbanization, labor migration, and changing gender roles have influenced the dynamics marital life in the area. Infertility is only one of the reasons that lead to

---

14. Setel et al., "Men's Perspectives," 12.
15. Nasimiyu-Wasike, "Polygamy," 101–18; Kanyoro, *Introducing Feminist Cultural Hermeneutics*, 86.

marital instability. This research has given four model narratives of infertile marriages. In chapter 5 the empirical findings will be discussed more theoretically, in the larger context of marriage in a transitional patriarchal community.

5

Life of Childless Couples in Machame

Construction of Social Identity in a Changing Society

Transition of Social Identifications

THREE THEORETICAL VIEWPOINTS WERE selected from the data of this study as being essential for the interpretation of childlessness in Machame. Social identity, shame and guilt, as well as coping were discovered in each model narrative. Each of these viewpoints assists in analyzing the narratives of childlessness in the Chagga community, and they are connected with one another. Social identity helps to analyze the relationship of a childless person within her/his community. The theoretical discussion about shame and guilt is needed in order to analyze the feelings of the childless person within her/his community. Coping is central when dealing with deviant behavior, as childlessness is understood to be, in a society where infertility is not a voluntary choice. These theoretical viewpoints have helped to interpret the more abstract meanings of the narrated life stories.

Identity is a widely studied concept in postmodern research. The concentration in recent years has been on personal identity. Narrative researchers have concentrated on autobiographies and, through them, the identity construction process.[1]

Erik Erikson defined personal identity as a "persistent sameness within oneself."[2] Erikson's definition includes an idea of sameness and is concentrated within oneself. Erikson criticized the traditional psychoanalytic method in that it cannot grasp identity because it has not developed terms to conceptualize the environment.[3] He noticed the need to define identity in connection with the environment, but his concentration was still, however, within oneself. Erikson's definition is not enough in the African context, so I turned to anthropology to find a definition that would work

---

1. See for example Holstein and Gubrium, *Self We Live By*, 105–6.
2. Erikson, *Identity*, 22–24, 45–50.
3. Ibid., 24.

in a Chagga context. According to Anita Jacobson-Widding, identity refers to sameness or distinction, and this is something we ascribe to other people as well as to something we experience within about ourselves.[4] Paul Ricoeur makes a similar distinction in his description of personal identity as sameness and selfhood.[5]

The concentration on sameness is useful in the Chagga context where identity is constructed in connection to other people. In a collective culture, identity is not a question of a single individual; the community is involved in the identity construction process. Von Bülow defines identity among the Chagga as being continuously constructed and transformed within a discursive process involving ethnic and religious discourses.[6] The concentration on selfhood is essential as a Chagga has his/her personal identity in the midst of the collective culture. Even though identity is constructed in relationship with others, the individuality of a person is recognized.[7]

The strong focus on the study of personal identity has its opponents in the Western context. The first social identity theory was formulated in 1970s, in the department of social psychology at the University of Bristol, as a rejection of individualism.[8] This so-called "Bristol school" formulated a second social identity theory which concentrated on self-categorization.[9] Both theories share in their definition that notion that individuals define themselves in terms of their social group membership.[10]

The social identity theory is well suited for use in analyzing empirical data from Africa because it does not presuppose Western individualism.[11] Younger Bristol social psychologists Michael Hogg and Dominic Abrams continue to analyze the social identity perspective. Their intention was not to add a new theory, but to integrate a comprehensive exposition of the social identity approach.[12] Their focus is primarily on the concept of the social identity rather than personal identity; in other words, they do not concentrate mainly on an individual's behavior, but instead on group behavior. Hogg and Abrams explain how an individual becomes a member of a community and how his/her social identity is developed depending

---

4. See Jacobson-Widding, *Chapungu*, 33.
5. Ricoeur, *Oneself as Another*, 116.
6. Bülow, "Power, Prestige," 3.
7. F. Shoo, "Tanzania," 102.
8. See Turner, foreword in *Social Identifications*, x–xi.
9. See ibid., xi.
10. Turner, foreword in *Social Identifications*, xi.
11. Hogg and Abrams, *Social Identifications*, 13.
12. Ibid., xiii.

on the group.¹³ They further claim that social identity mediates the dialectical relationship between society and the individual.¹⁴

The model narratives of childless couples reveal that childlessness is essentially a socially constructed reality in Machame. Medically diagnosed infertility is not a central issue in the discourse of childlessness in the Chagga context. The social nature of the problem poses a threat to couples' shared realities in a transitional society. The awareness that a person does not have children has consequences for the social identity among the Chagga.¹⁵

The approach of Hogg and Abrams concentrates more on social identifications than on social identity as such. They claim that the central question is about how people identify with a group and what the consequences are of such identification. They further define that social identity contains social identifications, which are self-descriptions deriving from membership in social categories such as nationality, sex, race, and occupation.¹⁶

Paul Ricoeur clarifies the relationship between identity and identifications in his definition: "The identity of a person or a community is made up of these identifications with values, norms, ideals, models, and heroes, in which the person or the community recognizes itself."¹⁷ Many identifications together construct the social identity of a person.

In a Chagga community, social identity is more salient than personal identity in self-conception because of the communal nature of the African culture. Social identities of childless persons in Kilimanjaro may vary. Some of them draw their identifications mainly from the Chagga tradition, others rely more on Lutheran teachings, while yet others refer mostly to modern influences. Van Bülow claims that identities among the Chagga are often interwoven in very complex ways.¹⁸

We have already defined the three cultural categories of *kienyeji, kikristo,* and *kisasa* in the introduction of this study, and have evaluated the influences of these cultural categories in the four model narratives. These narratives reveal that the new cultural categories do not displace the old patriarchal category, but rather all categories influence the construction of social identity in Kilimanjaro.

According to Hogg and Abrams, the above situation is such that one of the social categories tends to become more relevant to an individual than

13. Ibid., 25, 218.
14. Ibid., 26.
15. Miall, "Stigma," 270.
16. Hogg and Abrams, *Social Identifications*, 2, 25.
17. Ricoeur, *Oneself as Another*, 121.
18. Bülow, "Power, Prestige," 3.

other available categories depending on the relevant information available to her/him.[19] Hogg and Abrams maintain that people derive their identity in great part from the social categories to which they belong. Individuals belong to many different social categories and, therefore, potentially have a repertoire of many different identities to draw upon.[20]

Christian practices are no longer understood as modern and new. The cultural category *kikristo* relates to the historic churches, such as the Lutheran church in Machame, and are understood to have been part of the culture for a long time. Established Christianity is communal in character when everybody belongs to the same church in a rural village. The findings of this study reveal that charismatic Christianity cannot be grouped under the traditional *kikristo*, but should be under the category of *kisasa*, with the other modern phenomena. Charismatic Christianity is more common in the urban areas and contains aspects of modern individualism. The urban situation is more pluralistic, and new forms of Christianity are more easily accepted in towns than in rural Kilimanjaro. The reason for grouping charismatic Christianity under modern phenomena is neither theological nor geographical, but is a question of self-interpretation. The Chagga themselves interpret charismatic Christianity as a modern phenomenon that does not belong to traditional Chagga society.[21]

Chagga Christians purport that they are modern; however, the decisions that profoundly affect their lives reveal a close identification with traditional beliefs and practices. On one hand, *kienyeji* is labeled as backward compared to the modern, urban life style. On the other hand, in many community affairs, for example in marriage agreements, *kienyeji* is treated as an important cultural category.

Language is another important indicator of social identity in the multilingual Kilimanjaro area. The traditional language identity in the studied communities is the Chagga language, especially its Machame dialect. The Chagga language is used in families in the rural community, and the liturgy of the rural parish is in *Kimachame*.[22] The use of *Kimachame* is clearly diminishing; the younger generation does not speak it any longer. The national language, Swahili, is the language of urban families and the urban parish. Many urban parishioners use also English terms in their interviews to indicate how educated and modern they are. Interestingly, charismatic

---

19. Hogg and Abrams, *Social Identifications*, 25.
20. Ibid., 19.
21. A. Vähäkangas, "Responses to Prayer Healing," 161–65; Lugazia, "Charismatic Movements."
22. McGuire, *Religion, the Social Context*, 4.

Christianity uses many English terms as a way to denote how modern it is. The big evangelical meetings are called "crusades" in Swahili, and many charismatic Christians, even uneducated ones who do not speak fluent English, greet each with "praise the Lord." The transition in language identity is from the traditional ethnic language to the modern national Swahili language. This seems to indicate that the elderly people in Machame tend to rely more on the *kienyeji* category in connection to the language identity while the younger parishioners tend to rely on *kisasa*.

Jorge Larrain's analysis of cultural identity is useful when considering language identity in Kilimanjaro. Larrain describes cultural identity as being made and remade within available practices and relationships and existing symbols and ideas. Larrain points to the importance of different cultural institutions in the process of producing some public versions of cultural identity. These public versions then influence the way people see themselves and the way they act.[23] Among the institutions that influence the cultural identity, Larrain emphasizes the church.

The Lutheran church has strongly influenced the cultural identity of people in Kilimanjaro. It has strengthened the language identity by using the vernacular *Kimachame* in hymns and in liturgy.[24] Through the work of Lutheran missionaries in the area, the vernacular received its written form and its value as an accepted, official language. The influence of the church in Machame is wider than merely the influence of using the vernacular in church life. The Leipzig missionaries had the idea of *Volkskirche*, a communal people's church, as their missionary goal.[25] This missionary aim resulted in a strongly communal Christianity in all Lutheran areas of Kilimanjaro.

The Lutheran church in Kilimanjaro is strongly a Chagga church. Many aspects from the Chagga culture were transferred to the Christian church, but not all of them. Some aspects, especially the ancestral sacrifices and some of the rituals connected with the Chagga life cycle, faced disapproval from the Northern Diocese. One of these practices understood to be problematic to Lutheran Christians is the after-death memorial feasts. Aaron Urio's analyses that the Lutheran Christians seem to stand in two worlds, trying to follow both the Chagga and the Christian traditions, when they continue to conduct after-death memorial feasts even though

---

23. Larrain, *Ideology & Cultural Identity*, 163.
24. Hogg and Abrams, *Social Identifications*, 196.
25. Hasu, *Desire and Death*, 114–27; Shao, *Bruno Guttmann's Missionary Method*, 59–93.

the Northern Diocese strongly teaches against them.[26] Urio claims that the unclear relationship between traditional and Christian practices will continue to bring problems to the Lutheran Christians. He does not directly use the terms *kikristo* and *kienyeji*, but his analysis contains the idea of these two cultural categories.[27] Shao analyses the relationship between gospel and culture in the history of the Northern Diocese. According to Shao, the first bishop of the Northern Diocese, Stefano R. Moshi, had great appreciation for the African culture.[28] This study has revealed that the third contributing category, *kisasa*, makes the situation in contemporary Chagga society even more difficult.

Three cultural categories, *kienyeji*, *kikristo*, and *kisasa*, influence in various, even contradicting ways, the construction of male and female identities in Machame. The construction of male identity is discussed in the following section.

Male Identity in the Chagga Community

The relationship between fertility and social identity is essential in Kilimanjaro in the construction of both male and female identities. I shall first discuss the construction of male identity in Chaggaland. Those men who are suspected of being infertile seem to have difficulties in finding suitable social identifications and in constructing their social identity.

Table 8 evaluates the life stories of the four Chagga men who have lived in childless marriages. The focus of this table is on those factors that influence the construction process of the male identity in Machame. These four men are given titles to indicate the main message of their life story. Yeremia is the monogamist, he is the only model man who became committed to his marital union. Yakobo is the deserter who chose to separate from his official wife. Nehemiah lives in a formal polygynous marriage. Filipo is the "modern man" who does not live in a traditional polygynous situation, but chooses both to live with his official wife and to have a concubine. Filipo's title is a translation from Swahili, and it shows his interest in modern things.

---

26. Urio, *Concept of Memory*, 7.
27. Ibid., 7–8.
28. Shao, *Bruno Guttmann's Missionary Method*, 131–33; Howard and Millard, *Hunger and Shame*.

Table 8: Construction of Male Identity of Men of Model Narratives

Indicator of Male Identity	Yeremia, the Monogamist	Yakobo, the Deserter	Nehemiah, the Polygynist	Filipo, the "Modern Man"
Financial support	Supports Martha	Supported Raheli	Supports both Sarah and Neema	Supports both Blandina and Upendo
Place of living	Lives with Martha	Abandoned Leah stayed only with Raheli	Lived with both Sarah and Neema	Lives with Upendo but visits Blandina regularly
Male capacity proven or not?	No biological children	Children with Raheli	Children with Neema	Daughters with Blandina, sons with Upendo
Relationship to natal family	Invited a family meeting together with Martha	Advice from his parents and friends to desert Leah	His family accepted polygynous marriage	Family not involved in the decision
Building of a house	A house in an urban area	A house in village and another in town	Traditional huts for both of his wives	A house in the village
Work history	Teacher	Migrant laborer	Farmer	Migrant laborer
Status and wealth	Well off and valued	No longer well off and no longer valued	A valued elder	Well off and valued
Relationship to the Lutheran parish	Active parishioner	Still under church discipline	No longer under church discipline	Under church discipline

Financial support is an important indicator of male identity in Kilimanjaro. A traditional husband supports his wife/wives financially, at least to some degree if not providing all basic commodities. During the interviews several people pointed to Leah's financial assistance to Yakobo as an indicator of Yakobo's unclear male identity. Financial support is an indicator of power. A wife's financial support to her husband is interpreted in the Chagga community as revealing female dominance over male authority. The traditional role division among the Chagga has been that the wife is the provider of food in the family, but the husband is the provider of cash. Power relations have been essential to male identity. The social system of the Chagga society has preserved an excellent structural setting for a man to exercise his authority.[29] In such an authoritarian community, when a wife, even a former one, takes on the role of supporting the husband financially, it presents a new role division and exercises new values.

In the traditional Chagga community, wives reproduce the patriclan, meaning that the children always live with the paternal family. This traditional patrilocal situation is seen in the model narrative of formal polygyny, and in the model narrative of informal polygyny in the case of children of the first wife. In the urban, modern situation, children do not always live with their paternal family, as is seen in the model narratives of chapters 4 and 5.

There is a clear difference between traditional values on the upper slopes of the mountain in rural Kilimanjaro and those of the urban setting on the lower slopes of the mountain. This clear distinction between rural and urban life is seen in the interviews, and many informants, especially in the rural parish, maintain that life in the towns is immoral and corrupt.[30] Most of the model men have lived in towns, and this has clearly influenced their lifestyle. According to the analysis of the community, these men are suspected to have lived immoral lives in the towns.

We can evaluate the urban-rural difference in Kilimanjaro using concepts from the social identity theory. Recent research has found that in collective cultures, people construct a context-specific group norm from shared information. This norm can be called a group prototype, which describes beliefs, attitudes, feelings, and behaviors which bring the group closer together.[31] The traditional Chagga culture gave a normative group prototype to the members of the community. The situation in a changing Chagga community is not, however, as stable and coherent any longer. Only in the rural villages does the shared group prototype set norms to bring the group together. In towns and in villages closer to towns, the

---

29. Swantz, *Women in Development*, 79–88.
30. See also Haram, *"Women out of Sight"*, 210–11.
31. Terry et al., "Attitude-Behaviour Relations," 72.

situation is more pluralistic and the normative role of the community is much weaker.

Childlessness stigmatizes Chagga men as being impotent and therefore lacking the male capacity. The story of the committed union is the only one in which the male capacity was not publicly proven, and this seems to be one of the reasons why the husband, Yeremia, was suspected to be infertile. The assumption is that if he had not been infertile he certainly would have proven his male capacity by showing that he could beget children outside the family. An important part of male identity in Kilimanjaro is to be a father. In the African context, proving male capacity, as fatherhood is interpreted, is essential to the male identity. Dorthe von Bülow claims that fatherhood is an important part of maleness among the Chagga, although not the most important aspect.[32]

The strong traditional pressure of fatherhood contradicts the teachings of the Lutheran church about lifelong marriage and faithfulness to one's spouse. Childlessness is such a strong stigma in the Chagga community that it seems only the most devoted Christians do not search for a child outside of marriage. The traditional pressure of fatherhood makes childlessness a serious pastoral problem in the Northern Diocese, even though cases of infertility are not especially common.

The building of one's own house is a crucial male responsibility in Kilimanjaro. An adult Chagga male should build his own house, preferably in the village. Men who have migrated in towns are also expected to build their houses in the villages. The building of a house indicates wealth, another important value in the Chagga society. Wealth is an indicator of social status, and the male independent spirit in Kilimanjaro. Losing a house or living in a house that is in bad condition is a mark of shortcoming for a person's status in the community. Building a house on a plot of land in the family farm indicates a man's position in the family. This house is meant to be a reminder for a man working in town that his real home is in the village. To own a house in the village, even a simple one, reminds a man that there are demands of his inheritance later on. Having a house in the patrilocal homestead also shows the continuation of lineage and links to the ancestors. The land around the homestead continues to be part of the true identity of a Chagga man. The Chagga call these special lands by the term *kihamba*, which is a banana-coffee grove surrounding the homestead.[33]

32. Bülow, "Power, Prestige," 7.
33. Ibid., 8; Hasu, *Desire and Death*, 478–83.

In traditional Chagga society, warriorhood and leadership within the age group and the clan system have long been central for the construction of male identity.[34] The important setting of male identity was not only in the home but especially in the larger community. In contemporary society warriorhood is no longer central, but the qualities it represents, bravery and success, are still respected.

The leadership in the clan system is an important indicator of one's status in the community. The clan leaders are the ones consulted for various problems, and they are respected in the larger village community as well, not only in their own clan. Not every man grows into a position of authority in the contemporary society.[35] The position of authority in the contemporary Chagga society depends on personal achievements.

Wealth is a major contributor to high status in Chagga community, however, it is not the only way to gain status. Nehemiah is a poor peasant yet remains valued in the community because of his good moral behavior. Yakobo has financial difficulties, and neither his family life nor his life history provides him a respected place in the village community. Philip Setel shows that some occupations are more valued than others in contemporary Kilimanjaro. According to Setel, farming is understood, both in the traditional and in the Christian sense, to be honest and tiring work. Other occupations, such as being a business man or petty trader, are not valued as much in the Chagga community.[36]

The discussion in this section has revealed that construction of the male identity relies strongly on *kienyeji* cultural influences. The construction of the female identity includes more influences from various cultural categories, which will be discussed in the following section.

Female Identity in a Changing African Family

The setting of the female life stories is both at home and in the church. To be free to roam around in the larger community does not give a Chagga woman a respected status. The church and the Chagga community encourage women to concentrate on their roles and duties within the family.

---

34. Bülow, "Power, Prestige," 7.
35. Howard and Millard, *Hunger and Shame*, 162.
36. Setel, "Social Context," 41.

Life of Childless Couples in Machame 121

Table 9: Construction of Female Identity of Four Childless Wives

Indicator of Female Identity	Martha, the Only Wife	Leah, the Separated Wife	Sarah, the First Wife	Mama Juliana, the Official Wife
Whose fault?	Infertile husband	Stigmatized to be infertile	Known to be infertile	Has only daughters
Mother identity	An adopted son	Foster children	A social mother to Neema's children	Four daughters
Work role	Farmer	Paid laborer	A peasant	A peasant
Relationship with her husband	Good	Separated	Good	Tension
Financial support	Is supported	Self-reliant	Is supported	Is supported
Relationship with in-laws	Good	Problems	Good	Problems
Place to live	Urban setting, far from in-laws	Builds her own house	Lives in her own hut	Lives in Filipo's house next to in-laws
Role in the church	Active parishioner	A church elder	An active parishioner	A church elder
Burial place	Not revealed, most probably with Yeremia	Wants to be buried in the churchyard of the rural parish	Was buried in Nehemiah's homestead	Wants to be buried in Filipo's homestead

The cultural categories of *kisasa* and *kikristo* seem to influence the construction of female identity in Machame. The traditional influence, *kienyeji*, seems to be a frame of reference that is not as central in formulating female identity among childless women in Machame. However, the strong stress on motherhood and the need to have at least foster children to safeguard one's respectability reveal a connection to the Chagga traditions. The Chagga community, which influences the process of identity construction, stresses the *kienyeji* category, and through the community childless women are influenced by the traditions.

The life stories in the four model narratives reveal that marriage gives a woman a proper social identity. An unmarried woman is always called a girl and is not given equal respect in the community. A wife is a respected person in the community, but if she does not have a child something is lacking in her fulfillment of the female role.

Motherhood is an essential part of womanhood in Machame, and the crisis of infertility hinders the formulation of female identity. Von Bülow claims that motherhood is a summary of femaleness among the Chagga.[37] An important part of the identity of being a mother in Kilimanjaro is the new name a mother gets after the birth of her first child. Among the four women in the model narratives, Mama Juliana was the only one called by the name of her firstborn daughter; the others are referred to as a wife of somebody. Without motherhood, a woman sees herself as lacking something so fundamental that her very personhood is at stake. Being a mother means being a whole human being with a normal social identity and self-concept. Patriarchal society places motherhood above all other female role expectations and identities.[38]

It seems that the wives who experienced infertility were seen as failing in their normal role. This failure was so significant that is was treated as a challenge to their womanhood. In order to build strong female identity, the childless wives had to foster or adopt children, and thus become social mothers who are qualified to be treated as mothers in the community.

The identity of a woman depends strongly on men in the patriarchal Chagga society in Kilimanjaro. A woman is called somebody's daughter, somebody's wife, or somebody's mother. Her identity is predominantly communal, and this is why the social identification theory is especially important when analyzing women's identities in Tanzania.[39]

Leah was the only self-reliant childless wife among the four first wives of the model narratives. The others have husbands who support them at least partly. Financial support in Kilimanjaro is understood to be connected to the sexual rights of a husband. Leah's self reliance shows that her separation from Yakobo is also sexual separation. Financial self-reliance

37. Bülow "Power, Prestige," 7.
38. Inhorn, *Infertility and Patriarchy*, 56–57, 229.
39. Swantz, *Religious and Magical Rites*, 54.

indicates strong modern behavior, with a new kind of gender role that can be considered to belong to *kisasa* cultural category.

A woman's role in the parish is not only an indicator of interest in faith but also a way to achieve social status and strengthen her social identity. Chagga women are active churchgoers and all four first wives in the narrated life stories stressed the role of the church in their lives. An active role in the church has been important for the self-esteem of these women. Von Bülow analyses the role of women's groups in the church in regard to Chagga women's identity and shows that activities in the church are an accepted channel to leadership and improvement of living standards.[40]

The proper place for burial in the Chagga society is either the husband's homestead or the church yard, which are indications of an accepted female identity in the community. The husband's compound is the proper place for a woman to be buried, but if there are problems, such as the bride wealth having not been paid or the wife not having children, a woman cannot be placed there. Whereas the desired burial place would not be the first indicator of female identity in a Western society, African women in a changing society need to know where they will be buried. Only young girls are buried at their parents' homestead.[41]

Male and female identities are constructed in the community. The locations of these identities differ. The male identity is constructed in relationship to the larger Chagga society, but the female identity is constructed in the family.

Father Travels, Mother Stays at Home

An old Chagga proverb defines the father as the one who travels and the mother as the one who stays at home. The terms are used to indicate, once again, how a husband and a wife are always called father and mother in the Chagga community.[42] This proverb could not have been constructed to point to the couple only, as the Chagga have an understanding that a family consists always of parents and children. Tuulikki Pietilä writes on expected female behavior: "this positive immobility is expressed as staying, remaining, and living (*kukaa/kuishi*), which connotes fertility and continuity, and is revealed in 'cool' peacefulness."[43] A similar gender difference of location, as referred to in the proverb, is seen between the processes of

40. Bülow, "Power, Prestige," 12.
41. Hasu, *Desire and Death*, 478–82.
42. Rev. Anna Makyao, in her speech in a meeting of woman theologians in the ELCT on November 27, 2000.
43. Pietilä, *Gossip, Markets and Gender*, 261.

constructing social identities in Kilimanjaro. Indicators of the male identity are understood to be those things men do in the community, e.g., work history and other things discussed earlier. Female social identity is traditionally centered on the home, which strongly influences the construction of female identity among the Chagga women.

The above cited Chagga proverb could be interpreted to indicate the sexual freedom of a Chagga man to seek a child outside of wedlock. Thus, the proverb seems to allow a man the freedom to "travel" in order to have a child, but the wife should stay loyal at home. Even in the case of an infertile husband a wife was expected to stay at home. The men of the patriarchal family were supposed to help her, and she is not to travel in order to find a child.

Chagga women, especially those living in the patrilocal residence, find support in their problems from neighbors and the church community. Their own families and childhood friends often live far away. Chagga men who live in their home villages are able to search and find support from their natal families. The patrilocal practice is one of the reasons why women search for help from the Christian community or in an urban setting, from modern values. Rural men construct their identities in connection with *kienyeji*; many are also open to modern ideas, *kisasa*, but not especially in their marriages.

Traditional Chagga culture is collective, and its normative control is very strong as can be seen from the male narratives. The modern lifestyle is more individualistic and does not contain as strong a normative control. The traditional Chagga culture controlled female sexuality with strong behavioral norms. The church, through the practice of church discipline, tries to control male sexuality in contemporary Chagga community. Church discipline also controls female sexuality; for example, a large number of female parishioners are under church discipline because of premarital pregnancies.

The Northern Diocese has taken a role to control the behavior of its parishioners. This type of role is possible either in small church communities or in collective communities such as the Chagga community. In villages the Chagga culture seems to control the behavior of members of the community. In towns the situation is changing so that people are no longer under normative but under "attitudinal control," using the terms of David Trafimow who studied the relationship between private and collective self-concepts. Trafimow, a social psychologist building his theory partly from the social identity theory, showed that people in collective cultures are under normative control.[44]

Those women such as Leah who need to act against the traditional role expectations seem to construct their identity partly from the traditional male characteristics. They no longer follow the traditional advice of the proverb regarding the suitable locations for each gender. These women are not always able to stay in the African family, as is the case of a separated wife who no longer has a marital home to take care of. Unclear social identifications, as we have seen in the discussion in connection of constructing male and female identities in contemporary Kilimanjaro, makes it difficult for childless couples to find their own social identities. Self-disclosure is a respected adult behavior of both husbands and wives in Chagga marriages. The following section deals with the effects of this traditional behavior on childless marriages.

Shame and Guilt in the Lives of Childless Couples

Shame as a Violation of Identity

The previous section reveals that unclear social identification brings problems to an individual in contemporary Chagga community. In order to interpret the feelings of childless couples and the attitudes of the community towards them, I searched for a theoretical framework that would consider questions of identity as well.

The concepts of shame and guilt have been widely researched, especially among psychologists during recent years.[45] Psychologists, following the psychoanalytic tradition, have focused their analysis on the ego and superego, where the focus is on the individual. These studies recognize the importance of relationship experiences, particularly in the family, but do not consider the individual as a member of his/her wider community.[46] The psychoanalytic tradition does not deal much with social identity, which is central to the discussion about shame and guilt in Kilimanjaro.

Kaufman, however, considers the impact of culture in connection with how an individual behaves under shame. According to Kaufman, experiences of identification produce culture. Cultural identifications develop through, for example, story telling, which in turn reveals community

---

44. Trafimow, "Theory of Attitudes," 48, 51–55.
45. Kaufman, *Psychology of Shame*; Tangney, "Shame and Guilt"; Baumeister et al., "Interpersonal Aspects of Guilt"; Scheff, "Conflict in Family Systems"; Wallbott and Scherer, "Cultural Determinants."
46. Kaufman, *Psychology of Shame*, 24–25.

values as well as taboos to the listeners. Among the cultural identifications, Kaufman recognizes religious identification as well.[47]

Pastoral research on shame and guilt recognizes the importance of the religious community as a source of identification. Among those involved in such research are two Lutheran theologians from the United States: Robert Albers and Brad Binau. The previously discussed psychologists, especially Gershen Kaufman, have influenced the analysis of both Albers and Binau.[48] They build on the work of the psychologists but rename many of the concepts to fit the theological discussion and terminology.

Robert Albers defines guilt as a violation of one's value system and shame as a violation of one's identity as a person.[49] The definitions of Albers are useful when evaluating the lives of childless couples in Machame. Shame, which violates identity, is crucial in a transitional society where the couple has to cope with many different changes in their relationship and in the living conditions. Failure to cope successfully with the challenge of childlessness leads to feelings of shame.[50]

Binau uses the basic distinction of Albers between shame and guilt and maintains that guilt makes us question our actions while shame makes us question ourselves as actors.[51] Binau links the discussion of shame and guilt to a broader theological discussion about the concepts of law and gospel. He sees shame as a possible experiential correlation to the law. Binau claims that shame and law have the characteristic of exposure in common. He refers to Luther's second use of law and maintains that both shame and law point to the fact that our relationship with God has been broken.[52] Binau's insightful comments about shame and disunion with God and human beings are very appropriate to the discussion about shame in Kilimanjaro.

Tanzanian Sylvester Kafunzile has analyzed shame in the Haya society and uses the distinction of Albers between discretionary shame and disgrace shame. According to Albers, discretionary shame protects the person's world from disintegration and is necessary for a healthy individual. Disgrace shame can be a painfully paralyzing and debilitating experience.[53] Kafunzile's interpretation is that shame has been imposed on the childless

---

47. Ibid., 44.
48. Binau, "When Shame," 110; Albers, *Shame*, 3.
49. Albers, *Shame*, 22.
50. Kaufman, *Psychology of Shame*, 16.
51. Binau, "When Shame," 95.
52. Binau, "Shame and the Human Predicament," 128, 139–40.
53. Albers, *Shame*, 12–13.

Haya women so strongly that it ruins their identity for life.[54] According to Kafunzile, the shame that ruins the identity of childless Haya women is disgrace shame, the harsh and painful shame which does not protect one's personality.

The community and the couple themselves expect a child to be born in a Chagga marriage. A childless marriage is a source of shame in a community that expects children in the marriage. In the Chagga culture, shame is interpreted to be an emotional response to falling short of the social norm. In other words, shame is the feeling that one does not correspond to the culturally defined behavior that is attached to a particular social role. Christian couples face strong demands from the Chagga community. If these expectations are not fulfilled soon enough, the self-esteem of both the husband and wife is at stake. Spouses are affected by shame in various ways because of the lack of a child in their marriage. Brad Binau includes a similar dimension of shame in his definition, for shame points to the fact that we have all fallen short of what was expected.[55]

Shame is difficult to define in the Chagga context because only those actions that become known outside the family are believed to cause shame.[56] The belief that unknown things do not exist results in the hiding of family secrets. Similarly, in Kaufman's analysis to feel shame is to feel that somebody has seen you with a problem.[57] In the discourse of childlessness among parishioners in the two parishes of this study, the word *siri*, secret, was recalled numerous times. The proper behavior of an adult person in Machame is to keep the secrets of the family.

The Chagga family teaches its youngsters in contemporary society about proper marital behavior, including the idea that family matters should not be revealed to outsiders.[58] Only marital problems that are widely known are openly discussed. Albers has similar findings of family secrets in the Western context. He maintains that if people do not express problems openly shame will remain hidden as a secret of the family.[59]

The Swahili word for shame, *aibu*, is commonly used in everyday discourse on morality and proper behavior. In the data of this research, *aibu* was connected more often to pregnancy outside of marriage than to the shame of being childless. Comments on childlessness, which included word *aibu*, discussed the harsh words used to insult the childless wife. The

54. Kafunzile, "Shame and Its Effects," 78.
55. Binau, "Shame and the Human Predicament," 129.
56. Welbourn, "Some Problems," 189.
57. Kaufman, *Psychology of Shame*, 17.
58. Urio, *Concept of Memory*, 64.
59. Albers, *Shame*, 81.

use of *aibu* in connection to the verbal abuse seems to confirm that shame is connected to these insults.⁶⁰

Result of Verbal Abuse—Shame or Guilt?

Childless wives have to face harsh insults in Machame. One third-person narrator, a female teacher in the urban parish, condensed the discussion about verbal abuse: "Especially mother-in-law and sisters-in-law say dirty words. They just are not afraid at all. You know, there is the shame of eyes. You discuss even behind but if you meet (insulters) then they might decide to blame openly. This is why they are called the Palestinians, because of their cruelty."

This woman is from another part of Kilimanjaro, Marangu, and she can more openly criticize the Machame women, even calling them Palestinians. But is the question of verbal abuse only connected to shame, or is it also related to guilt? I used the definition of Robert Albers in the previous section, which definedd shame as a violation of one's identity. Albers defines guilt as a behavioral violation of one's value system.⁶¹ Thus, guilt has to do with one's behavior, not oneself. Our question is thus: Is the verbal abuse focused on the behavior of a childless woman or on her essence as a person?

Table 10 lists and classifies some of the verbal abuse documented in the data of this research. These insults about the wife were either told to the husband or directly to the childless wife herself.

Table 10: Insults about Childless Wife

Classification	Insult in Swahili	English Translation
1. Useless wife	Wewe kazi yako ni kuja kujaza choo hapa.	Your work is to come and fill the toilet here.
2. Useless wife	Hana faida kwetu.	We do not get any use of her.
3. Useless wife	Limekuja kula bure.	It came to eat for free.
4. Family background problematic	Kwao lilikosa chakula.	There was no food at its parents' place.
5. Witchcraft accusation	Yeye ni mchawi.	She is a witch.

---

60. Tangney, "Shame and Guilt," 114.
61. Albers, *Shame*, 22.

6. Misbehavior	Alipokuwa kijana alitumia madawa mengi sana.	When she was a teenager she used a lot of medicines (contraceptives).
7. Misbehavior	Ametoa mimba sana.	She did many abortions.

Insults were mainly told in third-person narratives, many of which were repeated many times during the interviews. These insults are only a few examples of the large variety of harsh words recalled during the interviews. Personal life stories included some of the insults, but generally the first-person narrators did not want to recall them. As one of the informants explained, "In the Chagga culture those who have problems do not want to discuss them, others will comment on these problems." These open insults at first seem to place shame on childless wives, but the different types of insults contain suspicions that the childless wife is guilty of something.

The first three insults indicate that the young wife is useless, showing that she does not belong in the patriarchal family. The nature of these insults is strongly patriarchal and stresses the importance of patriarchal and patrilocal family. The wife has an instrumental role in the traditional Chagga family. Reproduction is her main duty and through reproduction she can gain respected status. One reason behind these insults seems to be that the women of patriarchal family try to get the childless wife to decide to leave so they do not have to return all of the bride wealth, as was the case in the model narrative of desertion. The weak structural position of women makes them dependent upon other women in their patrilocal family. A conflict among sisters-in-law further weakens the position of a childless wife.[62]

Through insults, the women of a patriarchal family want to teach a young wife her role in the new family. The young wife, who in rural community moves to her husband's homestead, has to learn to adjust to new practices. An important part of this new role is the mother's role. If the young wife does not conceive soon enough, the women of the patriarchal family start insulting her. The blame of guilty actions is heavily balanced against the sociologically weaker generation, the newly married couple, and especially the woman.[63]

In Chagga society, women are expected to adjust to their new homes and to tolerate the situation there. Most of the interviewees in Kilimanjaro

62. Howard and Millard, *Hunger and Shame*, 148.
63. Raum, *Chaga Childhood*, 100.

hold the traditional point of view and only a few interviewees questioned the practice of insults. Various African theologians have discussed the situation of a young wife in the patriarchal family. Useful for the ongoing study is Mercy Amba Oduyoye's analysis of the situation of a young wife. She criticizes John S. Mbiti's patriarchal interpretation that it is the duty of the young wife to adjust. Oduyoye's feminist point of view is that the young wife should not have to adjust to every situation and should not tolerate everything in her new family.[64]

The language of the third and fourth insult (Table 10) treats a childless wife as a thing that has not done what was expected of it. The language used in these insults is extremely harsh. Placing the wife in the *ji/ma* class instead of using a personal pronoun indicates a hard criticism against her. In normal Swahili discourse, the verb is never conjugated according to the *ji/ma* noun class in connection with a human being except for the purpose of insulting. One of the connotations of the *ji/ma* class is to refer to something dirty and abnormal.[65]

The fourth insult is an example of those verbal abuses that blame the natal family of the daughter-in-law. The insult includes an idea that there was a poor financial situation in the natal home of the daughter-in-law. This type of situation is shameful among the Chagga, who connect financial abilities to the good upbringing of a child. Another reason for this insult regarding the lack of proper food is that it contains an explanation for the reason for her infertility. The daughter-in-law did not get enough nutritious food in her natal home, and as a result her reproductive capacity is low. Many of the insults clearly point to the problems in her childhood home and to the parents of childless wives, who should feel responsible for finding a cure for their daughters.

The fifth insult includes a witchcraft accusation; either the childless wife herself is accused of being a witch or somebody else is accused of bewitching her.[66] In the Chagga community, witchcraft is interpreted as being connected to misbehavior. It is, however, a little unclear whose misbehavior is supposed to have caused the infertility. In some cases it is claimed to be that the infertile woman is a witch herself, in other cases somebody else is accused of bewitching the infertile wife. According to the findings of Howard and Millard, when people in the same lineage find themselves in conflict they use various forms of spiritual harm. The notion

---

64. Oduyoye, "Critique of Mbiti's View," 351; Mbiti, *Love and Marriage*, 86–87.
65. Harjula, *God and Sun*.
66. Kafunzile, "Shame and Its Effects," 72.

that curse or sorcery can cause a woman's sterility is part of everyday life in Kilimanjaro.[67]

The last two insults in Table 10 place shame onto infertile women, but they also imply that guilt is connected to the case. These types of insults, which seem to be increasingly common in the contemporary Chagga society, blame the young wife for sexual misbehaviors, such as abortions.[68] Individual moral responsibility and guilt thus seem to be connected in the discourse of childlessness.

According to my data, childlessness seems to be more often related to beliefs of being cursed than to witchcraft. Grandmothers are those who are accused of cursing their granddaughters. If not grandmothers, then sisters-in-law are suspected to be behind the curse. Discussion about the difference between a curse and witchcraft reveals that it is connected to relationships between women on both sides of families. Sally Falk Moore argues, based on her field research in eastern Kilimanjaro as early as the 1960s, that the competition between the wives of brothers is indirectly a competition for land.[69] The lack of male offspring has serious effects on inheritance in Machame. In the contemporary community, the scarcity of land has decreased the pressure on land, but competition inside the family remains and contributes to the verbal abuse of childless wives.

The connection between sterility and carrying a curse makes a childless person feared in the community. Many informants recall some childless wives from their childhood community who were feared by the children. This fear of a curse on a childless wife is not only related to children. Childless wives are feared, but at the same time abused verbally. However, they may also be treated respectfully because of the fear of their curse. Those who are allowed to abuse a childless wife are the women of patriarchal family who seem to be already afraid that they have received a curse within the family. Others in the community try to avoid the curse, so they treat an infertile wife with respect.

Harjula's findings on guilt and curses are a helpful theoretical tool in analyzing the discussion about verbal abuse, which is part of the search for the reason behind childlessness in Machame. Raimo Harjula analyses guilt in connection to social relations among the Meru of northern Tanzania, an ethnic group that is closely related to the Chagga of Machame and who share similar traditions and beliefs. In Harjula's definition, guilt and curse are connected when looking for the reason for sickness. Harjula claims

---

67. Howard and Millard, *Hunger and Shame*, 154–56.
68. Silberschmidt, "*Women Forget*," 166.
69. Moore, "Selection for Failure."

that guilt is a communal feeling.[70] He says that whose guilt is connected to a curse depends on the case, but according to his findings, the guilt in most cases is connected to the guilt of the sick person.[71]

The insults of childless wives support Harjula's findings. It seems that the women of the patriarchal family lay insults on the childless wife because they feel that she is guilty of not conceiving. Through the insults, they tell the surrounding community it is her fault that their brother or son does not have children in his marriage. My discussions with parishioners in the two parishes reveal that insults place shame on childless wives and are used because childlessness is interpreted as revealing acts of misbehavior. Misfortunes in the Chagga context are understood to be the result of misbehaviors.[72]

Unclear social identifications make the feelings of shame and guilt more complicated in Machame. A curse is suspected in a situation where an individual does not have a good relationship in the community. Reconciliation of such relationships in the community helps to solve some of the shameful situations.

The extremely harsh language used regarding women who do not conceive brings shame on the stigmatized wife. Noteworthy is that the patrilineal community safeguards the man so that he is not insulted as openly as the woman.[73] The patrilocal system of residence has partly contributed to the unequal mocking of spouses. The social system of the Chagga society has emphasized man's control and superiority in the family and in the larger community as well.[74] The husband is the one who lives further away from his in-laws and is thus not usually insulted. Childlessness is not openly discussed in Machame, but my data clearly indicates that these insults are both very open and strong. Childless wives have a hard time when coping with the bad words. The collective culture of the Chagga has contributed to the way shame and guilt are interpreted in the community. Chagga people seem to experience more shame than guilt.[75] In addition to these immediate and visible effects of shame and guilt, my study reveals some less visible effects, which are discussed in the following subsections.

---

70. Harjula, *Syyllisyys, sairaus ja ihminen*, 75–97.
71. Ibid.
72. Howard and Millard, *Hunger and Shame*, 155.
73. Raum, *Chaga Childhood*, 76.
74. Swantz, *Women in Development*, 81.
75. Wallbott and Scherer, "Cultural Determinants," 469–70.

Dynamics of Honor-Shame

In the previous section we discussed the concepts of shame and guilt as revealed in verbal abuse. *Heshima*, honor, is a more frequently used concept than these in the discourse of childlessness among Lutheran parishioners. *Heshima* is connected to correct moral behavior, and in the data of this research it is mainly related to female sexual behavior. Honor is worth more than the value of a person in her own eyes, and especially in the eyes of society. Honor is the opposite of guilt. It is something one should have in order not to feel shame within the community.

Heshima is a wider concept than the English word "honor." *Heshima* can also be translated to mean respect and dignity. It is interpreted to be an important female behavior, but it is not very frequently connected to male behavior among active Christians in Kilimanjaro. A husband's behavior does not necessarily have to follow the Christian moral code because, again, the *kienyeji* category is more important for male *heshima*. Men in Kilimanjaro seem to earn more respect for the greater number of women and children they have. Thus, *heshima,* in connection to female behavior, seems to refer more to dignity, and in connection to male behavior it seems to be a mark of respect in the eyes of the community. Female behavior is seen to be home centered and male behavior community oriented.

Shame is more than a feeling of an individual in a communal Chagga culture. Women, who bear the family's honor through their respected sexual behavior, are the protectors against family shame. Childlessness poses shame on the natal family of a childless wife, but it also affects the life of a patriarchal family. Honor and shame are especially crucial elements in rural Tanzania where face to face relations are dominant.[76] The childless couples living in urban Kilimanjaro do not face shame as much as those who live in the villages.

Albers defines dishonor as a shame dynamic. He maintains that dishonor has to do with being stripped of a sense of dignity and integrity. The result of dishonor, according to Albers, is a horrible humiliation.[77] Only those deeds which are openly known bring dishonor to an individual in the Chagga community. The fear of being cut off from the family and the larger community is a great threat in Machame. Binau has similar findings in a Western context. He says that shame implies abandonment and the threat of being treated as an outsider.[78]

---

76. Silberschmidt, *"Women Forget,"* 166.
77. Albers, *Shame*, 47.
78. Binau, "Shame and the Human Predicament," 132.

The shame of childlessness is a lifelong stigma, as was seen in the narrative of desertion. The separated wife could not remarry. One of the interviewees explained that because she was stigmatized as being infertile it is not possible for her to be remarried. Chagga men expect a child from a marriage and would, therefore, not marry a woman who is known to be infertile.

The stigma of childlessness indicates a second dynamic of shame, which, according to Albers, is a sense of feeling defective.[79] A childless person is often described with the word *kasoro*, which can be translated as either "defect" or "fault." *Kasoro* also includes the idea that something is missing; a person who is described to be *kasoro* is not a whole person. A central issue in all the narrated life stories was trying to find whose fault childlessness was. The use of *kasoro* reveals that a childless person is interpreted to be physically defective. Albers similarly claims that any kind of physical disability may result in feeling "different."[80] The issue for the Chagga community is not only that an individual would feel different from others, but that others would label her/him to be physically disabled and not a whole person.

The above discussion reveals that shame is mainly a burden to women in Machame. Men face shame through church discipline, as we have seen in all of the narratives of this study. But what is actually the situation in the studied parishes? Do men feel shame at being excommunicated?

Excommunication seems to be a lesser source of shame for Chagga men than remaining childless.[81] The traditional pressure of fatherhood, the *kienyeji* cultural category, is thus seen again to be a greater burden for Chagga men than the Christian moral code and its control through church discipline. Excommunication does not seem to be a great problem for Chagga men in the twenty-first century. Even the pastors in both of the study parishes hesitated during interviews with the practice of church discipline. They expressed their concern that church discipline does not give them tools to control their parishioners. Also, those childless men interviewed and observed seemed not to stress the influence of church discipline to the decisions of their life. Church discipline was a more powerful way to control the commitment of Lutheran Christians in the traditional society that was more collective than the contemporary and more individualistic Chagga community.

---

79. Albers, *Shame*, 49.
80. Ibid.
81. Munga, *Uamsho*, 309.

F. B. Welbourn discusses the relationship between shame and guilt in the Ugandan context in the 1960s. He argues that African cultures are shame cultures in which becoming a Christian was a response to shame rather than claiming salvation from guilt. Welbourn continued to analyze the effects of shame culture in the life of Ganda men, and says that men officially accepted the taboos imposed by the missionaries until their traditions were offended, at which point they were ready to be excommunicated.[82] Excommunication was not a big threat for these Ganda men, who wanted to become Christians in order not to be left out of the community in a time when most Gandas converted to Christianity.

Binau's distinction between shame and guilt helps us to see why excommunication is a lesser shame than childlessness for men in contemporary Machame. Binau states that guilt focuses on actions, whereas shame focuses on identity.[83] Fatherhood is an important part of male identity in Machame. When searching for a child outside of marriage, a Chagga man does not seem to feel the guilt of his action, or at least he does not show it to others in the community. The greater shame for these Chagga men seems to be if other men look down on them for not fathering children.

Urbanization has further influenced the behavior of Chagga men to such a point that morality has become an individualized issue. The old controls of Chagga community, which were not very strict for men, do not restrict the behavior of those men who have migrated into town.[84] Shame and guilt, which are communal feelings in Machame, have a different effect on those couples who live in a village than on to those who live in an urban setting.

Discourse involving shame, guilt, and honor in the studied parishes reveals that the relationship between spouses is not expected to be equal. *Aibu* and *heshima* are connected to female moral behavior, which, in a patriarchal Chagga society, is controlled by men. Good moral behavior in Chagga women is a question of honor and social value. The power of shame disturbs the life of childless couples who need to defend themselves against the burden of shame.

Defending against Shame

The shame of childlessness produces an intolerable degree of discomfort in the lives of childless wives. Lutheran parishioners in Kilimanjaro defend themselves in various ways, most of the time unconsciously, against the

---

82. Welbourn, "Some Problems," 191.
83. Binau, "Shame and the Human Predicament," 132.
84. Setel, "Social Context," 57.

shame of childlessness. Albers names different ways of defending against shame: perfectionism, self-righteousness, power and control through disguised manipulation, blaming, martyr complex, and withdrawal and isolation.[85] In the analysis below I evaluate how these different ways of defense are used in Machame. Self-righteousness and blaming were used jointly in the female narratives. The martyr complex was not found in the data, thus only five different defense mechanisms are analyzed.

A childless person who tries to live a perfect life wants to eliminate any possibility of criticism. The separated wife is a good example of a person who wants to do everything as well as possible. Even the language used in her personal narrative reveals her perfectionism as was discussed in chapter four. Perfectionism as a defense mechanism is hard for a person to maintain for very long. The value of a person who tries to be perfect is always dependent upon what others say or think about her/him.[86]

In the first-person narratives nobody admitted that doctors would have found a physical reason for their infertility. Even the first wife of the model narrative of formal polygyny, who had had a surgical treatment, explained the situation as God's decree, not with a medical explanation. While medical examinations are not up to date in Tanzania, these denials seem to reveal that those stigmatized by infertility do not want to admit their problem. Many times the physical problem was identified, and third-person narrators seemed to have knowledge of it. People in Kilimanjaro seem to use denial of infertility as a defense mechanism against being stigmatized as permanently infertile.

Interviewed parishioners explained how a shame-based person acts in a Chagga society. Many explained that childless wives like to hide and are not socially active in the community. Withdrawal and isolation seems to be a defense mechanism of younger childless wives. In all the model narratives of childless wives, the tendency to isolate oneself was seen in a desire to hide or escape, which indicates feelings of shame.[87] Later in life these women tend to become more active in their communities. Some withdrawal is also seen in the life of a committed husband, especially when he is unwilling to discuss his infertility crisis with others. Generally, however, withdrawal seems to be a more feminine defense mechanism in Machame. Chagga men are expected to be more socially active and involved in the community affairs, even though they would like to cover up their shame.

---

85. Albers, *Shame*, 69–84.
86. Ibid., 70–71.
87. Tangney, "Shame and Guilt," 116.

Their active participation in the life of their local Lutheran parish seems to be the uniting component in the life stories of women in this study. Only one of the childless men is an active parishioner. This active participation can be seen partly as the support of the faith community for a childless individual, and partly as an attempt by the childless individual's to compensate for lack of status in the community. Religion seems to become a defense against the feeling of shame. Power and control through disguised manipulation is seen in many of the narratives. It is often the motive for the serving as church elders. The status of a church elder seems to be more important than the function the role serves.

The narratives of childless wives indicate a discontinuity in a story regarding the accusations against young girls who have had abortions. Childless wives defend themselves against their own shame by insulting others, especially those who do not have the status of being a married wife. Blame and self-righteousness are both connected in these narratives. The view of Albers that one way of defending oneself against shame is to put others down seems to agree with the data of this study.[88]

The above discussed defense mechanisms are utilized as strategies for survival. Defenses against the shame of childlessness are used mainly reactively and without any proper plan to cope with the problem. The shame of childlessness, which violates one's identity, requires a planned tension management through the use of either individual or united coping strategies that act against the demands of the variety of stressors. The stressors of childless marriages are more closely examined in the following section.

Tension Management of Childless Couples

Psychosocial Stressors of Childless Chagga Marriages

The life of childless couples contains verbal abuse and shame, as we have analyzed in the previous section. The early years of marriage are especially hard for a young couple. Childlessness is understood to be a form of deviant behavior in the Chagga society, and so these individuals have to learn to cope with it and to find their place in society. Childlessness is a difficult social situation, and without different coping strategies it is difficult to find one's own place in the community.[89]

Coping is an umbrella term that covers several life cycle factors. Coping consists of making certain general assumptions about one's ability to influence the course of one's life and one's capacity to reach specific and

---

88. Albers, *Shame*, 73; Tangney "Shame and Guilt," 124.
89. Mgalla and Boerma, "Discourse of Infertility," 197–98.

generalized goals. Various scholars, mainly psychologists, have contributed to the theoretical discussion about coping.

According to Susan Folkman, coping refers to cognitive and behavioral efforts to master, reduce, or tolerate the internal and/or external demands that are created by stressful situations. Folkman further claims that coping refers to efforts to manage demands, regardless of the success of those efforts. Coping helps a person to manage stress even though the difficult situation may remain unchanged.[90]

Folkman defines two types of coping based on the primary function: "emotion-focused coping" and "problem-focused coping." The former is a type of coping in which the regulation of emotions or distress is central, while the latter concentrates on the management of the problem that is causing the distress.[91] Coping with childlessness follows the latter function. The couples in Kilimanjaro have a visible problem both in their own understanding and in the eyes of the community. This problem that causes distress to the childless individuals needs management.

The starting point for coping research is the concentration on the postmodern individual, for whom the ideal is a lifelong process of identity construction. In coping theories it is presupposed that an individual has freedom of choice. It is assumed that the community may partly limit this freedom but does not control it completely.[92] Due to the emphasis on individual freedom of choice, many coping theories or models are better suited for Western, individualistic societies than for collective African cultures. In spite of the limited usefulness of Western coping theories, the concept of coping is useful in analyzing the life of childless couples in Machame. On the basis of their background, childless individuals belong to their collective culture. However, because childlessness is considered as deviant behavior, the Chagga community treats these people partly as outsiders. As a result of this, the childless people need emotion-focused coping due to their suffering from partial ostracism.

A medical sociologist, Aaron Antonovsky, concentrates his theory on how people manage to stay well in difficult life situations. His theory does not only concentrate on the individual level, but he recognizes an individual as part of the community, and he is especially interested in how the institutional roles in a society produce the strong feeling of coherence.[93] This makes his theory a valuable tool for evaluating the findings of this study.

90. Folkman,"Personal Control," 843.
91. Ibid., 844.
92. Järvikoski, "Sisäinen elämänhallinta," 45.
93. Antonovsky, *Health, Stress and Coping*, 25; *Unraveling the Mystery*.

Antonovsky identifies three components of the sense of coherence: comprehensibility, manageability, and meaningfulness. In other words, persons with a strong sense of coherence have abilities of comprehension and management and have found meaning in their life. Antonovsky calls his theory the salutogenic model of health.[94] The person with a strong sense of self and a firm identity will be one with a strong sense of coherence. A person with a weak self will latch onto a given identity. Such a person has a rigid sense of coherence, and his/her perceptions of high comprehensibility, manageability, and meaningfulness allow for no substitutions.[95] Because the identity is given, and not personally constructed, any change affecting it represents danger of losing the ready-given identity.

Tension management is the process of dealing with tension. Stressors place a load on people. How people deal with this tension is central in Antonovsky's theory. He uses the word "stress" only if this tension is not successfully overcome.[96]

Antonovsky focuses on health, not sickness, in formulating his theory. Here he differs from Lazarus and Folkman who see stressors as being a threat to a person. Lazarus and Folkman do not make a distinguish between stress and tension, which is central to Antonovsky's sense of coherence theory.[97] In a difficult life situation, a person gets help through different coping strategies. A coping strategy is an overall plan of action for overcoming stressors. It is a plan for behavior, not the behavior that eventually results from coping with the stressor.[98]

A stressor is defined as a demand made by one's internal or external environment. People differ in the extent to which they can contain and cope with these stressors. One type of stressor is psychosocial, that is, connected to both one's psyche and social relationships.[99] Psychosocial stressors are the most apparent in the case of those dealing with childlessness in a Chagga community. They are inherent in the whole life span of infertile couples. These stressors are also mainly external, due to the Chagga culture in which childlessness is not treated as only the problem of an individual couple but as the concern of the whole African family, as seen in the model narratives of this study. Three partly-contradiction cultural categories apply stress to infertile marriages.

---

94. Antonovsky, *Unraveling the Mystery*, 16.
95. Ibid., 26.
96. Antonovsky *Health, Stress and Coping*, 3; *Unraveling the Mystery*, 130–35.
97. Raitasalo, "Aaron Antonovskyn," 61.
98. Antonovsky, *Health, Stress and Coping*, 111–112.
99. Ibid., 72, 79, 82, 85, 105.

Modern influences are seen in the changing roles of spouses, especially in the urban setting. Labour migration has strongly affected the marital life of three out of four couples. The model narrative of a committed union elaborates the good influences of the more individual aspects of an urban life style, which, in this example, contributed to the well being of the childless couple.

The fear of HIV/AIDS, resulting partly from urbanization because of the loosened control of sexual behavior in an urban setting, is one of the psychosocial stressors of infertile marriages. The fear of AIDS affects all marriages in contemporary Kilimanjaro, but especially infertile marriages, where there is an additional pressure to have children out of marriage. Even committed Christians cannot trust their Christian spouses completely. The traditional pressure to have children seems many times stronger than one's Christian moral values.

In an urban situation, the nuclear family is becoming increasingly important in supporting elderly people. Those elderly people who do not have their own children are supported, to some extent, by their larger family, but they do not usually receive as good care as those who have their own children. Childless couples have doubts about whether there will be someone to take care of them when they are old, as was seen in the model narrative of a committed union. Through the adoption of a son the couple safeguarded their future.

Privatization of social relations and financial resources has led to a situation where one's own children are becoming an even more important source of support in old age. In the traditional Chagga society the entire Chagga family shared resources together, but in the contemporary society a nuclear family uses most of its income for its own household needs, even though it may still give some support to the less well-off members of the clan. Coping is more difficult in a transitional society; subcultures are changing, and this usually decreases the support of a community for an individual.

Chagga values can bring negative effects on the commitment and unity of Christian couples, as seen in all of the model narratives. One of the strongest external stressors of childless couples is family interference. All four childless marriages faced it. The role of mothers as sustainers of the Chagga traditions is revealed in all of the narratives. Patriarchal mothers seem eager to interfere in their sons' marriages. Family interference adds more stress to those couples living in the patrilocal homestead. In the urban situation there is less family interference.

The pressure to have biological children becomes more apparent in the adult relationships of spouses. All couples in the model narratives coped well with childlessness during their first years of marriage, but a clear change came approximately five years into their unions. In one case the period of crisis led to the strengthening of the marriage, in one case to separation, and in two cases it resulted in the addition of second wife.

The pressure for biological children results in a small number of adoptions in Kilimanjaro. There are many orphans that would be available for adoption, but few Chagga couples are willing to apply for an official adoption. Usually a child must be a blood relative because this type of fosterage is more acceptable than adoption.

The Northern Diocese and its parishes stress lifelong marriage and absolute monogamy. These demands are controlled through church discipline, as was frequently seen in the narratives. We have previously discussed that church discipline does not seem to cause much shame among parishioners in Kilimanjaro. It does, however, add stress to the childless spouses who, according to the church, have to obey the demands of their Lutheran parish. This pressure on the part of the church seems to be especially difficult for Chagga men, who have to deal with the additional communal pressure of contradicting the *kienyeji* category.

An individual's interpretation of the demands and pressures of a childless marriage regulates the coping process. Couples generally try to compensate for childlessness in other aspects in their lives. The tension management of psychosocial stressors is discussed in the following section.

Active or Passive Tension Management?

Childless marriages in Kilimanjaro have various psychosocial stressors, as discussed in the previous section. Christian couples have to cope with the demands of the family, the church, and the changing Tanzanian society by using various methods of tension management. Antonovsky measures tension management by the rapidity and completeness with which problems are resolved and tension dissipated.[100]

Couples in Kilimanjaro do not identify their marital problems openly, as was earlier discussed in connection to the shame-guilt-honor concepts. Also, tension management by childless couples is not dealt with openly; most of the time it does not include a carefully planned procedure. Some individuals and couples seem to work out their tension management

---

100. Ibid., 96.

better than others. However, active tension management seems to help couples to deal with childlessness and its effects within their life.

In order to cope with childlessness an individual has to have a balance between personal decisions and the expectations of the community. A person without strong self-esteem and a certain degree of autonomy cannot use active tension management in her or his life. Riihinen claims that the disabled are not given the responsibility of self-government in many societies. Included in Riihinen's disabled class are children and persons with severe mental illness or severe physical handicap.[101] In Chagga society, one could perhaps also include women with those who are not given the responsibility of self-government. Other aspects of autonomy, in addition to self-government, are self-identity and self-reliance. The only woman in the model narratives with a strong degree of autonomy was the deserted wife. She wanted to be self-governing and self-reliant as part of her active tension management process.

Passive defenses, such as blaming or withdrawing from social contacts, negatively affect the process of coping. Susan Folkman and Richard Lazarus call these passive defenses "primary appraisal." Primary appraisal is a situation in which a person's self-esteem is at stake and the feelings of shame are strong.[102]

The cultural value of keeping family secrets leads many childless Chagga couples to cope only passively with the stressors of this problem in their marriages. Antonovsky calls this "passive tension management." The use of defense mechanisms seems to reveal the influence of the *kienyeji* cultural category in the life of childless couples or individual childless spouses.

The process of coping with the strains of life happens both consciously and unconsciously, depending on an individual's capacities and self-esteem. Lazarus's colleague Susan Folkman terms the evaluation of coping resources as a "secondary appraisal" of the process of stress and coping. She defines secondary appraisal as the evaluation of coping resources, including physical, social, psychological, and material assets.[103] Secondary appraisal focuses on problem solving. The life stories of this research reveal that some of the couples and some individuals used more active tension management in their lives than others. Active coping seems to need more modern attitudes and a strong self-esteem to act against some of the taboos of the traditional Chagga society.

101. Riihinen, "Elämänhallinta-käsitteen," 18.
102. Folkman and Lazarus, "Coping and Emotion," 214.
103. Folkman, "Personal Control," 842.

But how can an individual reach secondary appraisal or, using Antonovsky's term, "proper coping?" The "general resource for resistance" concept (GRR) in Antonovsky's sense of coherence theory refers to characteristics that facilitate dealing with and overcoming a stressor.[104] According to Antonovsky, GRR are those resources that help active tension management. Two different types of GRRs are classified according to their origins. Outer GRRs are resources that deal with the stability of society, with the different role structures in the society, and with material resources. Inner GRRs deal with one's own capacities and life experiences. Antonovsky's scheme of inner and outer GRRs comes very close to the designation of inner and outer coping methods, which is used by many scholars writing on coping.[105] Table 11 compiles the inner and outer GRRs found in the model narratives.

The model narratives reveal that outer resources have contributed to the coping process of many childless couples in Machame. Access to money seems to be an important external GRR in the Chagga community. A strong financial position gives a person a more respected status in the community, as was revealed in the narrative of a committed union, whereas insufficient wealth is seen as a complete failure within the Chagga community, as discussed in the case of the deserting husband. Possession of housing also influences the coping possibilities. More flexible gender roles, as seen in the case of the separated wife, were seen as an important resource, along with a stable work situation. In those cases where there was unemployment or labor migration, this was seen to negatively influence the individual's coping process.

The model narratives reveal that education is an important internal resource for coping in contemporary Kilimanjaro, as was seen, for example, in connection to the committed husband. Various difficult life experiences, such as the childhood family situation, were seen as having a positive contribution to the coping process in the case of the deserted wife. Also, intelligence, a good variety of relationships, and various social roles were seen both in the narrative of a committed union and in the case of the deserted wife. These strengthened the childless person's role in the community and enabled the construction of strong self-esteem, which further contributed to more effective coping.

Inner and outer GRRs can enable a childless couple or an individual childless spouse to cope with the stresses of living in a Chagga community without a biological child. Many times there is not, however, a clear

---

104. Antonovsky, *Health, Stress and Coping*, 105.
105. Ibid., 106.

Table 11: Inner and Outer Resources of Childless Individuals

Outer Resources	Inner Resources
money	education
housing	life experience
flexible gender role	strong self esteem
physical strength	intelligence
stable work situation	social relationships and roles

distinction as to whether a resource is internal or external. Olavi Riihinen claims that evaluating the division between internal and external coping is often a bit problematic. He evaluates coping as the cooperation of both internal and external resources.[106]

Couple's Joint versus Individual Coping Strategies

The use of active tension management for overcoming the demands of the African family, changing society, and moral expectations of the Lutheran church indicates the use of coping strategies. Again, a coping strategy is, according to Antonovsky, an overall plan of action for overcoming stressors.[107] Antonovsky claims that the question is not which coping strategy is used, but how many are used and how flexible a person is in employing different strategies.[108] I would claim that, in the case of childless couples, the question is note merely about which coping strategies are used, but rather, are the strategies used to strengthen the marriage or to strengthen the self-esteem of only one of the spouses?

According to Antonovsky, coping strategies are always conducted in a historical-cultural and situational context.[109] Social change has led to changes in the roles of spouses. In a changing society marriage becomes more than just an institution for reproduction; the partnership dimension of the marriage also becomes quite important.

The various coping strategies used in the model narratives were discussed in the narrative chapters. The focus of this section is to analyze how these selected coping strategies were used.

---

106. Riihinen, "Elämänhallinta-käsitteen," 29–30.
107. Antonovsky, *Health, Stress and Coping*, 112.
108. Antonovsky, *Unraveling the Mystery*, 141.
109. Antonovsky, *Health, Stress and Coping*, 112.

Table 12: Individual and Joint Coping Strategies

Coping strategies used in agreement between the spouses	Coping strategies, used by one spouse only
adoption	fosterage
family meeting	separation
official polygyny as an agreement between spouses	children from "outside," no disclosure to the spouse
growing independence from patriarchal family	obedience to traditional values and listening to the advice of the patriarchal family
support of a faith community to a couple	support of the faith community only to one of the spouses

The narrative of the committed union reveals the strong united coping strategies used to strengthen the childless marriage. The common decision to adopt a son was an important coping strategy which helped to strengthen the marriage of the committed couple. The fosterage of children, as seen in the life story of the separated wife, was an individual coping strategy which helped a childless woman gain respected status in the Chagga community. The narrative of formal polygyny indicates how the couple proceeded together to make the decision to change their marriage from monogamous to polygynous. In the narrative of informal polygyny, the pursuit to bear a son without the knowledge of the official wife indicates an individual coping strategy.

The deserting husband followed the culturally accepted coping strategy of adding another wife in order to have children. The narrative of desertion, in chapter 3, does not reveal a single uniting coping strategy; instead it reveals the various individual coping strategies used by both spouses. A growing independence from the patriarchal family is also seen as a central coping strategy of a committed couple.

Obedience to the traditional values is seen to influence the variety of coping strategies in all other model narratives except in the case of the committed union. Obedience to the traditional values is more closely followed in the rural setting, where the whole Chagga family resides in the same homestead. Support from the faith community was seen in the model narrative of the committed union as a joint coping strategy and in other model narratives as a coping strategy for the childless wife. Support from of the faith community will be more closely discussed in the following section.

Support of Faith Community in Coping with Childlessness

The church community is seen to be an important support channel in coping with childlessness in Kilimanjaro. The faith community has been especially important for female parishioners. This seems to correspond the fact that the active Christians in the Lutheran parishes in Kilimanjaro are mostly women. The findings of von Bülow reveal that the church community offers regular and accepted social networks for Chagga women.[110] Women will lose their respect if they search for social networks from local pubs or other social places, but their husbands will usually accept the activities at the church, which are family and domestic oriented.

Antonovsky's sense of coherence theory maintains the idea that in many societies the control is located in a deity or in the hands of powerful others.[111] In Machame the role of church workers, especially that of the ordained pastors, is to control the life of their parishioners. Childless wives have found that when pastors control their husband's behavior, the faith community actually supports these women and their role in the family.

All four childless wives were active parishioners. Two of them were given the respected role of a church elder during the time of the interviews, and none of the first wives had ever been under church discipline. The church community supported all of them through various visits, prayers, and even finances during their time of infertility crisis. All these wives have used active tension management and have overcome the stage of isolation, which is the tendency of deeply shamed people, as has already been noted. According to Albers, the debilitating effects of shame are overcome only through social networks in a community.[112] Antonovsky similarly stresses the importance of a community. He claims that the social networks to which one is committed are a crucial generalized resistance resource.[113]

All the narratives of childless wives mentioned the important role of the church community and revealed the various activities these women regularly attended. The deserted wife was the only one who explained, in length, the role of prayer in her life. The others included prayer as a natural part of being in a faith community, even though they did not expound on

---

110. Bülow, "Power, Prestige," 12.
111. Antonovsky, *Health, Stress and Coping*, 155.
112. Albers, *Shame*, 106.
113. Antonovsky, *Health, Stress and Coping*, 116.

it. Albers discusses the community of faith as being essentially a community of prayer and mutual disclosure which is made possible by faith.[114]

The social identity theory stresses that in-group norms influence behavioral intentions only for those who identify strongly with the group membership.[115] The data of this study supports these findings. The only model husband whose behavior followed the behavioral teachings of the Lutheran church was also a committed Christian. All those model women who identified strongly with the church followed the norms of the church in their lives.

The church workers have to maintain a difficult balance between various cultural categories while searching for their own point of view on life and their spiritual work. Others rely more on the *kikristo* cultural category, many of whom are clearly following the official practices and values of the Lutheran church, but at the same time relying on both the *kisasa* and *kienyeji* cultural categories. There seems to be a trend among church workers to be more open to *kienyeji* than during earlier years. We could name those following this trend the "re-traditionalists."[116] Many Chagga theologians are proud of their roots and would like to use some traditional values in order to help their parishioners cope with contradicting social identifications.[117]

The parishioners seem to construct their identity somewhat from the *kikristo* cultural category and quite strongly from the *kienyeji* category, but modern influences are also contributing to the identity construction process of most of the parishioners. It is important to note that Christian, traditional, and modern influences all contribute to a person's behavior.

There is no united theology of marriage in the Northern Diocese. Many church workers stress how Christian marriage is a contract between husband and wife, and they further assert that children are only gifts given to a couple, not something they should either demand or take for granted. This "official" Christian teaching on the role of children in a Christian marriage is in contradiction with the traditional point of view where the family is understood to consist of parents and children. A husband and wife without children do not constitute a socially recognized unit within the traditional Chagga community. Most of the interviewees admit that

---

114. Albers, *Shame*, 106.
115. Terry et al., "Attitude-Behaviour Relations," 91.
116. Kerner, "Chaptering the Narrative."
117. Shao, *Bruno Gutmann's Missionary Method*; Urio, *Concept of Memory*; Malewo, *Pre-marital Counseling*.

children are not a requirement within a marriage, but, subconsciously, their desire is for children in all Chagga marriages.

Church workers and parishioners expressed the need for communal support for the childless couples. There seems to be a need for contextualized Christian counseling in the parish community. Such counseling should be holistic, uniting the various cultural categories in order to strengthen marital life within the community.

6

Sense of Coherence as Wholeness

African Wholeness and the Sense of Coherence

In many Tanzanian ethnic societies, among them the Machame, an adult is described as *mtu mzima*, a whole person.[1] This wholeness, *uzima*, refers to more than an individual's age and is a wider concept than the English word "wholeness" communicates. It can be translated to mean vitality, adulthood, completeness, energy, existence, maturity, and perfection. All of these definitions have been revealed in the model narratives of this study. *Uzima* is thus a central concept for interpreting childlessness in Machame.

A full adult is a person who has children, preferably through marriage, but single people with biological children are also considered to be adults. A childless person is, thus, not considered to be a whole person—he/she lacks something essential for wholeness as it is understood in the traditional African setting. In order to achieve wholeness, or at least to approach it, a person living under the stigma of childlessness has to find different coping strategies to be accepted within the community, as was seen in the previous chapter.

Aaron Antonovsky's sense of coherence model helps to interpret the Chagga understanding of wholeness. Antonovsky defines sense of coherence as "A global orientation that expresses the extent to which one has a pervasive, enduring though dynamic feeling of confidence that one's internal and external environments are predictable and that there is a high probability that things will work out as well as can reasonably be expected."[2] How people handle and cope with the demands of life largely depends on their sense of coherence. Antonovsky makes a clear distinction between sense of coherence and the psychological concept of ego identity. He maintains that ego identity refers to a picture one has of oneself, while

---

1. Mbiti, *Love and Marriage*, 11; Pobee, "Life and Peace," 17; M. Vähäkangas, "Ukristo, Uzima, na Ujamaa," 45–50.
2. Antonovsky, *Health, Stress and Coping*, 123.

sense of coherence refers instead to a picture of one's world. This world, of course, includes the self.[3]

Through this entire study we have examined the influence of three cultural categories leading to the construction of social identity in Kilimanjaro. In connection to the Christian life, we have to remember that the *kikristo* category refers to an imported Christian cultural framework derived mainly from the early missionaries; it is a foreign product in Kilimanjaro. *Kikristo* does not refer to Christian dogma, but to its cultural expression in the West. *Kikristo,* as it was brought to Kilimanjaro, contained many Western cultural aspects, among them ideas regarding what a proper Christian woman's place is in society and marriage. The aim of the Leipzig mission was not to bring their own culture to the Chagga people, but this intention was not preserved in all aspects; for example, while teaching on marriage the Leipzig missionaries followed German tradition and introduced the German scheme of the division of labor and the domestication of housewives in Christian families.[4]

Until this stage of the analysis, the discussion has been on the cultural categories. However, to proceed further one needs to elaborate Christian faith in relation to the cultural categories. I prefer not to use the term "Christian theology" because it usually refers to an academic form of theology that is also a product of Western intellectual development and is generally too abstract to describe the life situation in Africa.

The same tension Christians experience in their lives also influences their formulation of faith. The pastors and theologians in Kilimanjaro feel this tension when they try to take a stand on many of the practical issues related to the marriage of their parishioners. A frequent way to deal with these pastors has been to consider them as having a superficial or weak Christian faith, blaming their weakness as the cause the difficulties in formulating indigenous Christian practices in Kilimanjaro. This is, however, an outdated colonial idea.

South African theologian Manas Buthelezi's distinction between two approaches of theology assists in analyze the situation in the contemporary Chagga church. Buthelezi calls the first approach the ethnographical approach. Its focus is on the indigenous church structures and theology.[5] Buthelezi, however, criticizes this first approach as the way Westerners try to indigenize African theology. Buthelezi argues that in the ethnographical approach the person with an African worldview is missing, and that

---

3. Ibid., 110.
4. Hasu, *Desire and Death,* 114.
5. Buthelezi, "Toward Indigenous Theology," 56.

the African worldview is treated as if it were something static.[6] Buthelezi maintains, if we use the terms of this research, that the ethnographical approach concentrates mainly on the *kienyeji* category and tries to imply that African thinking exists today as it did in the traditional African society.

Buthelezi calls the second approach the anthropological approach. The point of departure for indigenous Christian faith is not an ethnographically reconstructed worldview, but relies on Africans themselves. The presupposition of the anthropological approach is that Africans, as God's children, are not to be an object of study. Buthelezi maintains that the only way to meet people's needs in contemporary Africa is to follow this second approach. According to Buthelezi, theology in Africa must reflect the life situation in which people find themselves. Contemporary Africans find themselves alienated from the wholeness of life. Buthelezi purports that the reason for this alienation is theological dishonesty.[7] Buthelezi thus links the anthropological approach to the search for wholeness of life.

Buthelezi's theological model helps to understand the search for wholeness in Kilimanjaro. The focus of the construction of indigenous faith is on the Chagga Christians, not on some church structures or on the reconstruction of a traditional Chagga worldview. While the focus is on Christians themselves, their search for identity is essentially on being Chagga who are Christians. In this search, the missionary brand of Christianity is no longer valid; there has to be a search for indigenous Chagga understandings of faith and Christian practice. I would be following the ethnographical approach if I, as a European theologian, started to point to which direction the Northern Diocese ought to continue in this process. The process of finding faith identity needs to follow the anthropological approach, and this can only be done by indigenous Chagga theologians. One of them, Aaron Urio, has gone far in this direction while searching out a contextual theology of the Holy Communion.

Musimbi Kanyoro claims that the African Christian lives in the dilemma of gospel and culture. Kanyoro sees a way out of this dilemma if we analyze both the personal and the communal experiences in religion and culture.[8] Both personal and communal experiences have to be considered in order to cope with childlessness in the Chagga community. Both the contemporary Christian practices and the Chagga traditions have to be considered. Kanyoro's model of the dilemma of gospel and culture is a reality in Kilimanjaro.

6. Ibid., 60, 65.
7. Ibid., 65, 69–70.
8. Kanyoro, *Introducing Feminist Cultural Hermeneutics*, 19.

Chagga Christians try to balance between two worlds because part of their tradition is not accepted in their diocese. Those traditions which are not accepted include, for example, memorial feasts for the departed, part of bride wealth transactions, consultation of diviners, and polygyny.[9] The Northern Diocese seems to follow a policy where there is a clear distinction between which is a Christian practice and what is not. The charismatic Christianity that came with the American missionaries starting in the 1960s has brought stronger pietistic regulations to the Northern Diocese; for example, the use of local beer in marriage transactions was not a problem to the Leipzig missionaries, but it is a problem to the Northern Diocese at the moment.[10] The idea of making a clear distinction between Christian and traditional practices seems to complicate the life of Christians in Kilimanjaro. Healey and Sybertz define this type of situation as a dualism and parallelism between Christianity and African traditional religion. They claim that if African Christians continue to maintain this distinction there will be no wholeness in their life. According to Healey and Sybertz, one holistic world is what is needed in the life of African Christians.[11] Andrew Kyomo illustrates the same need for uniting the traditions, while he claims that there is a need to build a bridge between African traditional religion and Christianity.[12]

The balancing between various social identifications seems to interrupt the wholeness of life among Chagga Christians. The strong regulations on which practices are interpreted to be Christian and which are not seem to confuse the Christians of the Northern Diocese. Yet these regulations have not stopped most of them from practicing, for example, ancestral sacrifices. Instead, these sacrifices are carried out in such a way that pastors and church elders do not know about them.

In an African context, Antonovsky's sense of coherence model, which seeks a picture of one's world as a whole and does not concentrate only on individual capacities of control, is an essential tool for analyzing coping strategies.

African Immortality versus Christian Immortality

Central concerns of childless parishioners in Machame are related to the problem of immortality. This is explicitly emphasized in the third-person narratives and implicitly revealed in the first-person life stories, as were

9. Urio, *Concept of Memory*, 7; Malewo, "Pastoral Counselling," 83.
10. Hasu, *Desire and Death*, 117–19.
11. Healey and Sybertz, *Towards an African Narrative Theology*, 293.
12. Kyomo, "Faith and Healing," 147–52.

discussed when analyzing the different burial plans for two of the first wives. African immortality, the requirement of the continuation of lineage, is thus seen to be a central theme in the lives of childless couples in Machame.

Various African scholars have explored the discussion about immortality in Africa. Aaron Urio has analyzed at length the concept of memory in the Chagga life cycle. According to Urio, those persons who leave no offspring behind are believed to be cut off from life here on earth and in the hereafter. People who do not have children are thus considered to be the most unfortunate of people because they will leave no memory behind them.[13] Urio's argument reveals the importance of community in the Chagga understanding of memory and immortality. A childless person is understood to be cut off from life after death, African immortality, and also from communal life here on earth.

Shoo stresses the value of children in Machame. He is convinced that people who have borne children do not die.[14] Shoo does not, however, discuss what happens to childless persons, nor does he consider how they are linked to African immortality. Urio and Shoo are both fathers themselves. For them it seems natural to stress the value of children in connection to African immortality.[15] They are both among those Chagga theologians who are open to the contextualization of Christian practices. These two Chagga theologians derive their analyses and interpretation from both *kienyeji* and *kikristo* cultural categories, and they continue to search for an indigenous Christian interpretation of faith which suits contemporary Chagga situation.

Mercy Amba Oduyoye, a feminist theologian from West Africa, discusses the other side of immortality. She confesses that she does not have children and discusses her own position in an African community as a childless wife. Oduyoye defines Christian immortality as an identity with and in Christ. According to Oduyoye, neither Christian nor African immortality requires individual physical reproduction to become visible.[16] Oduyoye and the deserted wife in the model narrative are both active African Christians and childless wives. They both derive their interpretation of immortality mainly from the *kikristo* category. Christian immortality is central for both of these African women. They both claim in their own way that the tradi-

13. Urio, *Concept of Memory*, 1035, 117–26; Moore, "Chagga of Kilimanjaro," 46–47.
14. Shoo, "Traditional African Marriage," 26.
15. Gutmann, *Frau bei den Wadschagga*, 583; Dundas, *Kilimanjaro*, 126.
16. Oduyoye, "Critiquie of Mbiti's View," 3, 347; Silberschmidt, *"Women Forget,"* 133, 148.

tional religious belief of "diffuse reincarnation," using the term of Geoffrey Parrinder, which depends on procreation, does not have to be the only way understand immortality in the African context.[17]

The concept of African wholeness requires African immortality. But what about Christian wholeness—can it be interpreted as requiring Christian immortality? It seems that only through a correct understanding of the resurrection of Christ that a person can be seen as complete in the eyes of God, and there alone can the identity crisis, shame, and coping problems of childless couples be solved. Binau claims that it is central to consider the eschatological dimension of coping with shame. According to Binau, Jesus's true identification with human experience must also address our future.[18] The shame of childlessness is closely linked to the shame of not producing new members for the clan, and therefore, not following the African view of immortality. The eschatological dimension, as stressed by Binau, is central to childless couples in Kilimanjaro. Christian immortality seems to replace the need for African immortality in the future plans of some childless individuals.

Oduyoye further claims that if marriage is defined as an experience of the love of God then the traditional stress on procreation does not become as central in African marriages. Oduyoye sees the African perspective on biological continuity as being anti-feminist.[19] If marriage is God-centered, then spouses rely on God in all their decisions, as well as during the hardships of marital life. Mbiti, who in other parts of his theological work stresses the importance of procreation for African marriage, claims, however, that a happily married life includes the wholeness of an individual.[20] In his definition of a successful marriage, Mbiti does not require procreation as a seal.

Among Chagga Christians, divine law has been mainly administered through church discipline as a way to control parishioners' moral behavior. The gospel has been mainly used in dealing with the earthly side. In the case of childlessness, the gospel, as a promise of the eschatological future of Christian immortality, seems to bring hope to some childless couples in Machame. Binau describes Christian wholeness when he claims that the divine law and gospel together result in a complete person. The overcom-

---

17. Oduyoye, "Feminist Theology," 170; Parrinder, *African Traditional Religion*, 136–40.
18. Binau, "When Shame," 109.
19. Oduyoye, "Critique of Mbiti's View," 342–47; "Feminist Theology," 171.
20. Mbiti, *Love and Marriage*, 221.

ing of shame and the silencing of the voice of the law depend entirely on healing.[21]

Healing as a Tool for Sense of Coherence

A pathway leading to successful coping in the African context is the concept of healing. Healing has been and still remains an important part of life in Africa. Healing in the African context is not limited to health, and a central element of it is the restoration to wholeness. In searching for healing, the need of the Chagga people is not only for medical treatment but also includes the liberation and restoration of their whole life.

The model narratives reveal two basic pathways for dealing with the crisis of childlessness. The first is more passive; the stressors are too strong and the self-esteem too weak when an individual does not have enough resources to cope with the problem actively. This first way leads to the use of passive defense mechanisms. The second way is when a couple or an individual has enough resources to use various coping strategies. This second way leads through healing to the restoration of one's identity and, finally, to wholeness.

The model life stories point to the fact that these two ways can be seen in an individual's or a couple's life story. In many cases the more passive way is used at an earlier stage of life. Later, life experiences strengthen ones resources in such a way that the use of active coping strategies becomes possible. This combination of using the passive path first and later finding the more active way of coping with childlessness is seen in the life story of the committed couple, and again in the life of the deserted wife.

The restoration to wholeness required a new understanding of immortality in both of these cases. The traditional way of dealing with the crisis in these example stories was found to be too limited. However, through uniting more modern aspects in their lives together with their Christian faith and support of their faith community, the healing and construction of strong self-esteem was possible in spite of their childlessness.

The process of being healed from shame involves a process of identity regrowth.[22] This identity regrowth is seen in the coping process of childless couples in Kilimanjaro. Restoration to wholeness was possible only in those cases where a childless person could construct a strong sense of self-esteem in spite of childlessness.

---

21. Binau, "Shame," 140–41.
22. Binau, "When Shame Is the Question," 110.

Jorma Laitinen analyzes shame and guilt in the light of the fall in Genesis. His main claim is that if we interpret the feelings of shame and guilt only through psychological theories, the whole picture of human life is not considered. God's grace without human contribution is essential when dealing with a shame-based person. According to Laitinen, creation already shows that God loves people, and this love is the only possibility for healing.[23] Albers has a similar conclusion to that of Laitinen. He claims that the Christian community can enable an individual to access wholeness and healing. The grace of acceptance and the love demonstrated by the Christian community creates a safe place for the healing process.[24]

Reconciliation in one's own community and to one's own past is an important part of wholeness in the Chagga community.[25] Social relations are essential to one's well-being. An old saying of African traditions defines the essentiality of social identity to one's personal identity: "I am because we are; and since we are, therefore I am."[26] It stresses the African worldview of community, in which the image and personality of an individual becomes important within the context of community.

In marital counseling in the Northern Diocese the needed communal aspect seems to be partly missing. A pastor of the rural parish has recently started to work together with clan elders to unite the support of family and church. She explained how effectively they had counseled one childless couple to stay together in spite of their problems. According to her, a big advantage of this communal counseling is that the African family is present during the counseling and will support the decisions of the uniting council. None of the interviewees of this study had received such communal Christian counseling, as it was only recently introduced into the rural parish.

African theologians have considered the possibility of supporting communal Christian marriages. Congolese professor Kasonga wa Kasonga calls such a counselling "African Christian palaver." According to him, African Christian palaver is a contemporary way of healing communal conflicts and crises. Wa Kasonga stresses the importance of community in solving marital conflicts in the contemporary situation. The biggest difference between the traditional elders' council and the African Christian palaver is that the latter considers Christ as the symbol of life. According to

---

23. Laitinen, *Syntiinlankeemus*.
24. Albers, *Shame*, 106, 133.
25. Harjula, *Syyllisyys, sairaus ja ihminen*, 95; "Curse as a Manifestation," 131.
26. Mbiti, *African Religions*, 108–9.

wa Kasonga, Christ is the only power able to transform our disintegrated lives through this counseling process.[27]

There is a need to motivate community members to cooperate in counseling. Nwachuku, from her experience in West Africa, does not support the Western form of individual counseling clinics, which deal with an individual couple's problems only. She claims that the involvement of the whole community is important, but she does not undervalue the central role of spouses in the counseling process either.[28] Mathias Mndeme has had similar experiences in Tanzania. According to him, healing and counseling should be done within a community, not outside it. Mndeme recommends special healing services to local Lutheran parishes, where the healing could be done in a basic Christian community.[29]

There are also those who see the dangers of traditional communal values for the marital life of couples in Kilimanjaro. Malewo analyses this problematic aspect of communality, whereby if married couples are more concerned about their family members than about their spouse it can cause damage to the couple's relationship.[30] The model narratives reveal that there should be a balance between the support of the clan and the independence of each couple in deciding their own way of life. Finding such balance is needed in every society, but it is especially needed in the rapidly changing society in Kilimanjaro. Restoration of wholeness is a strong need in Kilimanjaro. African Christians need their own identity as Africans and also as Christians. Modernization should not mean losing one's own identity and roots.

---

27. Kasonga, "African Christian Palaver," 59.
28. Nwachuku, "Perceptions on Family Counselling," 113.
29. Mndeme, "Healing Ministry," 174–80.
30. Malewo, *Pre-marital Counseling*, 43.

Conclusion

THE AIM OF THIS research was to find out how a childless Christian couple constructs its identity in a Chagga community. We noted that in a collective culture, identity is not only a concern of a single individual; the community is involved in the identity construction process. Through studying the four model narratives we have found out how difficult it is to construct both personal and social identities without a child. The findings of this study reveal that concentration on identity was crucial. The unclear social identifications have made the construction of social and personal identity difficult for the childless Christian couples.

The decision to use model narratives as opposed to using authentic life stories was predominantly an ethical decision. I did not want the interviewees, some of whom revealed their life secrets to an outsider for the first time, to suffer within the community because of their involvement in the research project. The final report uses model narratives and, in addition, contains authentic accounts from the interviews. This combination works in a convincing way to shed light on the identity construction of childless couples in Machame.

The model narratives of this study are not meant to be read as representatives of all possible types of childless marriages. Using typology, in my case model narrative, always generalizes the result. My aim has been to share some of the common types of narratives with my reader in order to offer a better understanding of my theoretical analysis and also to offer a possibility of finding alternative readings.

The data of this study consisted of both first- and third-person stories. This was well-suited for use in the model narrative approach. If I had used authentic life stories as such, the third person accounts would not have been needed because the focus would have been completely on the first-person experiences. The use of two types of stories made the analysis more demanding, but it also resulted in the model narratives, in which the aspect of community, so central in the African context, is also considered.

The communal aspect continues to be central among the Chagga, although the Chagga community is and has been for a long time, in transition. The greatest difference between the contemporary situation and the past is that the range of identities is expanding. In this changing situation the current study has classified three cultural categories which work side by side: *kienyeji*, traditional; *kikristo*, Christian; and *kisasa*, modern. We have used *kienyeji* to denote the Chagga traditions, the ethnic identity of the Chagga people. *Kikristo* has been used to refer to the imported Christian beliefs and practices of the early missionaries in the history of the Northern Diocese. Therefore, *kikristo* does not refer directly to the contemporary teachings of the Lutheran church in the Kilimanjaro area. *Kisasa* has been used to denote those cultural practices and beliefs that result from education, modernization, and urbanization in Kilimanjaro.

Especially in the urban situation people are left without the support of both religious and local communities. Hence, the normative role of communities, both church communities and clan ties, is breaking down. There is a need to find new ways to support and control parishioners in regard to their communal needs. The findings of the current study indicate that this new way should contain aspects of *kienyeji* and *kikristo*, which are respected cultural categories. Many people have very definite opinions about changes, especially about the urban way of life, which they feel to contain questionable practices. Other modern changes, such as education, are well accepted in Kilimanjaro.

Healing, reconciliation, and reconstruction are needed at the family level, especially in the marital life of the parishioners, as well as in the context of the wider community. The overcoming of shame depends entirely on healing. The shame of childlessness, which violates one's identity, requires planned tension management against the demands of a variety of stressors. The process of healing shame involves the regrowth of identity.

Wholeness refers to completeness and perfection in Kilimanjaro. A childless person is not considered to be a whole person; he/she lacks something essential for wholeness the way it is understood in the traditional Chagga setting. In order to achieve wholeness, or at least to approach it, a person living under the stigma of childlessness had to find various coping strategies to be accepted within the community. Restoration to wholeness was seen possible only in those cases where a childless person could construct a strong sense of self-esteem in spite of childlessness. Healing in the African context is not limited to health, and a central element in healing is the restoration of wholeness. Reconciliation in one's own community and to one's own past was seen to be an important part of wholeness in the Chagga community.

The findings of this research reveal, on one hand, that the life stories of childless couples are full of stress and difficulties. On the other hand, they reveal that many of the narrated life stories are actually stories of success. Some Christian couples and some spouses have learned through their difficult life experiences how to cope with their childlessness.

The most important part of life for infertile people was to find resources for coping and, through these resources, to actively use various coping strategies. The cultural value of keeping family secrets has, however, led many childless Chagga couples to use only passive tension management.

It was found that some coping strategies were used in agreement with spouses, while other strategies were used by one spouse only. Adoption was among the joint coping strategies. Narratives on adoption in both study parishes reveal that adoption is understood to be a problematic coping strategy in the Chagga context since an adopted child is not a blood relative. Without biological procreation one is considered completely cut off from the family, both in this life and in the hereafter. In the urban situation, the possibility of formal adoption seems to fit better as an acceptable coping strategy. The joint coping strategies were found to be used in order to strengthen the marriage, and among committed couples the partnership dimension of marriage seems to become more important.

Individual coping strategies used in the model narratives of this study included, for example, fosterage, separation, and seeking children outside marriage. Individual coping strategies were mainly used to help an individual spouse cope with childlessness. The use of individual coping strategies increased the distance between the spouses.

In a changing society coping has required a reconstruction of social identity that does not depend on only one of the cultural categories but relies on a combination of at least two of them. Identities shift in response to situational contexts. As a result, the multiple identities of a childless individual sometimes conflict with one another. Learning to combine various identities in a way that does not lead an individual into an inner conflict has been found to be essential for coping.

It seems that only through a correct understanding of the Christian concept of resurrection can the identity crisis, shame, and coping problems of childless couples be solved. Through salvation by the cross a person can be seen as complete in the eyes of God, and understanding this will enable a childless person to restore his/her identity. On the cross God himself suffered and was weak. The theology of the cross helps a childless couple to tolerate their problem. The Christian faith, which enables a childless couple or a childless spouse to trust in Christian immortality through salvation in Christ, was found to be an important part of the coping process in Kilimanjaro.

While analyzing the data of this study, I noticed that I had paid too little attention to one important aspect. During the group interviews some women in the urban parish stressed that bride wealth is no longer important among the Chagga. This comment persuaded me to leave out questions on bride wealth during the two phases of personal interviews. While writing the final report, I began to regret this decision.

The role of bride wealth as a bonding factor among the Chagga should be addressed in another study, preferably by a non-theologian. According to Hasu, the full customary bride wealth includes various banana beer celebrations.[1] The Northern Diocese does not accept the use of alcoholic drinks, therefore, parishioners would not reveal such practices to a pastor, or at least not admit that they have themselves followed them.

In the beginning of my study I focused only on childless women. Fortunately, I extended my scope to deal with Christian couples and also considered the male experience of childlessness. Unfortunately, the number of childless men interviewed in this study is limited. There is a need to conduct further study on marital coping among childless husbands in Kilimanjaro. To conduct such a study would not be easy because, as the results of this study reveal, childlessness poses an identity crisis especially for men in the Chagga community. As a result, men are not ready to discuss their experiences and are not willing to be interviewed. In spite of the small sample of childless men, I could identify the difficulties for constructing male identity.

The role of single mothers in the Northern Diocese has not yet been studied either. I collected some life stories of single mothers but did not use them in the current study. My aim is to use this data later to study the role of single mothers in the parish community. These women form a relatively large percentage of the parishioners in Kilimanjaro, but their role and their needs are not addressed in the parishes.

As was already discussed, there is a need to construct an indigenous Christian theology of marriage. Various studies, the current one among them, have focused on the situation of marriage in the African parishes, but so far there is no indigenous theology dealing with the issue.

---

1. Hasu, *Desire and Death*, 253–66.

APPENDIX A

Sample Interview Questions

THESE QUESTIONS WERE USED in an interview of a church worker in the urban parish on March 10, 2000. They have been translated from Swahili.

1. Would you explain the value of children in Machame?
2. If couples failed to have children,
    a. In old days, what did they do?
    b. Today, what do they do?
3. What is the role of parish in helping the childless couples of the community?
4. Why do many youngsters have their marriage blessed only after their first child is born?
5. What teachings on marriage do you have in your parish?
6. What do people say is the reason for childlessness?
7. What is your point of view? Is the problem of childlessness more common today than it used to be in the traditional society?
8. Do you know couples who do not have children? Could you explain about their life to me?
9. What is the role of a childless person in your parish? How are these married but childless people respected in your parish?
10. Are young people afraid of childlessness?
11. What teachings on the value of children in marriage are used during send-offs and weddings? Are there special songs or proverbs in Machame which talk about the value of children?

Appendix B

Direct Quotations in Swahili

Chapter 2

MARTHA: *Sasa mara ile ile nilipoolewa hivi. Baba yangu akaja. Akamwambia, wewe ukiwa kama umeoa mtoto wangu, mimi ninataka sahihi yako. Basi bwanangu akaweka sahihi na mimi nikaweka sahihi na baada ya hapo nikabaki naye sasa. Basi hapo hapo, nikabaki na huyo mume wangu hapa na mama mkwe wangu yupo X sikuweza kusikia maneno yoyote. Basi tukabaki hadi hapo tulipofunga ndoa na mume wangu. Wakati kulikuwa na mchungaji anahamishwa, akasema siwezi kuacha ndugu zangu wakiwa nje, basi akaturudisha kundini na kutufungisha ndoa. [. . .] Saa ile si aliweka sahihi mbele ya baba yangu? Sasa ile sahihi si akaweka tena mbele ya kanisa, angewezaje kunifukuza?*

AULI: *Tuliongea kuwa kama watu wanaongea kitu kibaya . . .*

MARTHA: *Mambo haya yapo ndiyo.*

AULI: *Na unafikiri ni kwa nini wanasema hivi?*

MARTHA: *Kwa muda uliokaa pale nyumbani na halafu wanakuona kuwa wewe siyo wa pale, lazima.*

AULI: *Hivyo wanaona kazi ya mama ni kuzaa?*

MARTHA: *Ndiyo.*

AULI: *Lakini siyo furaha tu, kupata mke kwa mtoto lakini wanaona ni muhimu pia kupata mtoto . . .*

MARTHA: *Wanaona ni furaha lakini azae.*

AULI: *Hivyo inakwenda pamoja.*

MARTHA: *Ndiyo.*

MARTHA: *Mimi na bwana wangu tulisubiri kwa amani lakini huko pembeni maneno maneno yalitokea.*

AULI: *Lakini maneno ni kutoka nje ya nyumba?*

MARTHA: *Nje ya nyumba ndiyo.*

AULI: *Lakini ni kutoka kwa familia au ni majirani tu?*

MARTHA: *Familia ndiyo mawifi. Maneno yalitokea lakini tuliyapunguza.*

AULI: *Unaonaje maneno haya ulihitaji kuwajibu au ulinyamaza tu kama ulisikia?*

MARTHA: *Walisema labda kwa mume wangu. Tukasuluhisha yakaisha.*

PASTOR: *Nikamwuliza, alikuwa anajisikiaje? Akasema alikuwa anajisikia vibaya sana. Kwa miaka yote amekaa na mke wake hawakuwahi kupata mtoto. Na huyo mmoja alisema, alitamka kweli siku hiyo akasema, "Hata kujiua niko tayari kujiua sasa." [. . .]*

AULI: *Hivyo kweli alisikia vibaya.*

PASTOR: *Alisikia kwamba . . . Afadhali niondoke duniani tu. Tena akasema, "Afadhali niende kwa Baba."*

PASTOR: *Lakini mpaka wewe mchungaji uwe tayari kwenda.*

AULI: *Mmh! Ndiyo. Siyo kwamba watakuja . . .*

PASTOR: *Hawatakuja kwako.*

AULI: *Kukuulizia?*

PASTOR: *Hapana, hawatakuja kwako.*

AULI: *Ni kazi ya mchungaji kuwatafuta?*

PASTOR: *Kuwatafuta. Kwa sababu they feel lonely, they feel desperate here, and in addition to that they that the society may be they have neglected them. [these words were said in English during the interview]. Sasa kwa hiyo wanatafuta mtu anaye watafuta. Na wala si mtu anaye . . . sio wao wanakwenda. Hawawezi kwenda. Wewe uende ujenge urafiki, basi na wao watakuja kwako.*

MARTHA: *Mimi nilishirikiana na mama mkwe wangu wala sikuona shida. Wala sijala kidonge. [. . .] Wengine wanatoa mimba, unafahamu?*

AULI: *Ndiyo.*

MARTHA: *Akitoa ile mimba utaona Mungu amekutunzia nini, haya wewe utakuwa hupati tena watoto.*

AULI: *Na unaonaje, hii ya kutoa mimba siku hizi ni kawaida au inatokea mara nyingi au?*

MARTHA: *Mara nyingi, watoto wa kike wanatoa mimba sana! Kule kutoa mimba utakuwa Mungu amekupatia yai moja au mawili, au unakuta Mungu alimpa kiumbe kimoja tu katika tumbo lake, je atakwenda kutoa wapi? Ni hao hao ndiyo wanokuwa shida kwa bwana zao.*

PARISHIONER: *Mume wa huyo mama, anakuwa mvumilivu, anavumilia asikate tamaa. Kwa sababu unakuta kwamba baba haoi mke wa pili wala haonyeshi chuki kwa mke wake. Wanavumiliana wote, wanavumiliana wote. Ingava mara nyingine yule mwanaume naye, anaweza kuwa analaumiwa na wazazi wake. Lakini hakati tamaa wala haonyeshi chuki.*

PARISHIONER: *Wanavumiliana na wanapendana na wanashirikiana, na hawajakata tamaa. Na ni watu wenye uchaji. [. . .] Moja walichofanya, wanashirikiana vizuri. Hakuna aliyemchoka mwenzake. Hawajaishi kwa kushindana.*

PARISHIONER: *Huwa haskiriki anapenda starehe sana.*

AULI: *Eeeh sawa. Hivyo hana shida yeye mwenyewe hata kama . . .*

PARISHIONER: *Hana shida hata kidogo.*

AULI: *Eee, hivyo haileti shida kwenda na wakina-mama wengine kama hajapata mtoto?*

PARISHIONER: *Haileti shida kabisa.*

YUPO *cheerful, happy kabisa huwezi ukatambua. Hali uliyomona nayo ni hiyo hiyo. Huwezi kumuona amesononeka, Akalemewa na ile hali ya kutokuwa na mtoto, Yupo . . . yupo ana-match na group kabisa. Hajachukua kama kilema, au kasoro. Anaona is alright na tena ni mwenyekiti wetu. Halafu na maana yake sasa ni mama mtaratibu sana. Mtaratibu, mchangamfu, Anapenda kushirikiana na wengine. Anaupendo, Anakauli nzuri. Sasa sifa zote anazo.*

Chapter 3

LEAH: *Nilijitunza katika usichana tangu utoto mpaka nilipoolewa. Kwa hiyo hilo ilinisaidia. Hakukuwepo na ile lawama, oo sijui labda wewe ulikuwa hivi, umeshatembea nje, ndiyo sababu huna mtoto. Labda ulishatoa mimba!*

AULI: *Na mume wako alijua hiyo?*

LEAH: *Ehee! Ndiyo yeye . . .*

AULI: *Kwamba ulikuwa na sifa nzuri?*

LEAH: *Ndiyo hiyo hicho kitu kwanza, ile kwamba nilipoolewa mimi nilikuwa sijafanya kitu chochote. [. . .] Kwa au katika . . . Ilinisaidia. Kujiamini kwangu mimi, hata mtu asingetaka kuniamini zaidi ingenisaidia. [. . .] Kwa hiyo sasa kujitunza usichana kunasaidia sana, huwezi kupata lawama aina yoyote. Na hata . . . na mimi pia kwenye ndoa yangu sikulalamika.*

LEAH: *Muda unazidi kwenda kwenda, zijapata mtoto. [. . .] Kujaribu kuishi hivyo . . . lakini sisi hatujagombana wala kuchukizana hata kidogo. Mpaka ilipokaribu miaka sita hivi! Mwaka wa saba ndiyo akaanza kuona kwamba . . . akaona mtoto haonekani . . .*

LEAH: *Sikupata shida, lakini shida, isipokuwa ni hiyo familia tu ya wazazi hao,*

WALIKUWA *wanaona kwamba kwa nini mtoto wao hajapata mtoto. Wanakuwa wanauliza tatizo ni nini? Kwa sababu, linaumiza sana mchungaji. . . .*

AULI: *Na hasa hao wote?*

LEAH: *Mama mkwe, mama mkwe na wale wasichana wake. [. . .]*

AULI: *Kwa upande wa familia yako?*

LEAH: *Familia yangu . . .*

AULI: *Hawajaona shida?*

LEAH: *Wanaona, lakini sasa unajua, wanabeba ule mzigo wangu kama wa kwao.*

PASTOR: *Kwa hiyo watu wanapotazama wanaona yeye alifanya vizuri. Kwa sababu inaonekana! Kama angebaki tu na huyo [. . .] huyo!Basi* leo angekufa hakuna watoto. Na hii ni mkosi. Kwenye jamii ya Kichaga. Hata Kiafrika pia. Ndoa bila watoto hiyo inahesabiwa haikukamilika.

EVANGELIST: *Bado walikuwa wanaona kwamba huyu mama ni mwaminifu, na mama ambaye ni mtaratibu. Hata walipoona hicho kitendo ambacho kilifanyika hivyo ni kwamba walishangaa wakasikitika. Wakaona kwamba, haikuwa vizuri. Na hata wengine wanakuwa wanaendelea kumlaumu. Huyu baba, wakamlaumu hata mdhamini kwa sababu ya kusimamia hata yeye.*

LEAH: *Walisema angesikiliza maneno ya mchungaji. Kwa sababu mchungaji alimwambia ni vizuri kuoa mke mwingine kama ulivyooa. Lakini ujue kwamba huyu ndiye mke wako wa kwanza. Na nyumba ni yake, Huwezi kumwabia ondoka . . . Hata kama ni kujenga, jengea pembeni. Au kama ni chumba, pataneni akupe chumba kimoja ukae na huyu mke mwingine. Lakini huyu nyumba yake, mwenye mji ndiye huyu. Lakini kama unaogopa ukamfukuze huyu ukachukue mke mwingine, Hujabarikiwa. [. . .]Akasema kama ni watoto, mletee huyu alee hao watoto. Ndiyo hivyo. [. . .] Mpe-mpe watoto hao awalee.*

LEAH: *Huwezi kujua Mungu amepangaje! Au kupitia mahali ni Mungu anapanga kwa maisha yako. Lakini kitu kikubwa ni kiasi cha mtu kumjua Mungu. [. . .]Kwa hiyo hata kile unachotaka kukifanya au unapotaka hivi ni kuomba. Ukimwomba Mungu, ukimgojea, Mungu anatenda.*

AULI: *Ndiyo. Na uliona kwamba kweli Mungu ana nguvu?*

LEAH: *Sana.*

AULI: *Hata wakati wa ugumu wa maisha,*

LEAH: *Wakati wa ugumu huo. [. . .] Hata wakati mwingine hata mchana, natumia muda wangu nasali. Jioni hivyo hivyo.*

PASTOR: *Hajarudi kundini kwa sababu bado hajampa mke wake haki. Kwa sababu tuna utaratibu hivi! Ikiwa mke wa kwanza amekosa watoto. Lakini yupo hai, sasa ili kuhalalisha ndoa ya huyo mwanamke wa pili, lazima kisheria avunje ndoa ya kwanza. Na baada ya kuvunja ndoa ya kwanza lazima ampe basi yule mke wa kwanza haki yake inayomwangukia. Amjengee nyumba mahali pake, na kihamba chake. Mahali ambapo anaweza kufanya shughuli zake, kama ana uwezo, mpaka Mungu atakapo muondoa katika ulimwengu.*

LEAH: *Kwa sababu unakuta ile group ya kuishi na wenzako, ni kufurahia maisha.*

AULI: *Ee ndiyo ndiyo. Ulipata msaada kutoka hawa vikundi vya akina mama na kwaya pia?*

LEAH: *Ndiyo. Ukiwa lonely sana, peke yako, inakuwa siyo vizuri. Lakini unapoungana na wengine, mnatoleana mawazo, mnafurahi, kubadilisha mawazo,*

AULI: *Na maombi pia?*

LEAH: *Na maombi yanasaidia.*

AULI: *Hivyo kwa mfano wakati wa miaka kwenye shida [. . .] Ulikuwa na akina-mama wengine na waliweza kukusaidia?*

LEAH: *Sasa. Ee sana. Wakina-mama wengine wamenisaidia sana. [. . .] Kitu ninachokiona kwamba ukiwa na tatizo, usilibebe kama ni kubwa sana. Au usitembee njiani, umebeba matatizo. Ishi sawa sawa kama watu wengine. Usibebe kila saa shida shida shida.*

LEAH: *Nimeshaweka bati, Lakini sasa bado milango, madirisha pia bado. Bado sana.*

AULI: *Ulianza lini kujenga nyumba?*

LEAH: *Nilianza ni kitu kidogo sana lakini kinagharimu hela nyingi.*

AULI: *Mmh! Naona unajitahidi sana, he-hee!*

LEAH: *Utafanyaje ndiyo maisha sasa kwa sababu gani, Kama pale nyumbani, Kaka yangu ana mke, ana watoto na wao wanakua. Niende pale, mtu anaona kama nina—umekuwa mzigo kwao, kwa ile familia.*

AULI: *Mmm unapenda kujitegemea?*

LEAH: *Eee ni vizuri kujitegemea, angalau kuwa mzigo mwepesi kwa ndugu zako. [. . .] Usi—unapokwenda pale unakuwa mzigo mzito kwao.*

AULI: *Ni furaha zaidi unapokwenda na unajitegemea?*

LEAH: *Eee unajitegemea, unakaa mahali pako naye akitaka anakuja pale kusalimia.*

LEAH: *Hapa ndipo ninapokaa na wengine, hapa na mtoto wa kaka yangu, na kaa na wa dada yangu, na nyumbani wakati wote, Nikiwa nili . . . kuna mwingine nilimlea tangu miaka miwili, mpaka sekondari, amemaliza, Sasa hivi yuko . . . mkubwa! Ameshaoa! Ana mke.*

AULI: *Ndiyo, na pamoja na mke anakuja kukuona?*

LEAH: *Kabisa. Yeye ni kama mtoto wangu.*

LEAH: *Hata yeye alikuja hapa sasa yeye akaanza kusema, Aliomba msamaha, Akaja tena kuomba msamaha . . . "Kama tunajua kwamba tulikoseana nini na nini." Mimi nikasema na mimi nishakusamehe siku nyingi wala sina kosa. Isipokuwa sasa nilimwambia kama sasa umeoa, una watoto. Ukiacha wale watoto . . . kuzaa siyo kazi, kazi ni kulea. Ni vizuri ungelea wale watoto.*

LEAH: *Kutafuta pa kuzikwa haitoshi. Ni wewe mwenyewe kwa – kwenye moyo wako, Uzungumze na Mungu wako, Ujitakase, Ili ukapate kuurithi ule uzima wa milele. Huu – huu mwili, Kuuzika mahali, unaweza ukazikwa mahali po pote. Lakini je? Ni nini nitakacho-fight, Ni kupata ule urithi wa Mungu, ambao Bwana ametutayarishia. Ambao kila mtu anahitajika autafute kwa bidii.*

AULI: *Kwamba kaburi siyo muhimu sivyo?*

LEAH: *Ndiyo. Ndiyo. Lakini zaidi sana niku-fight kujiandaa kwa kule maisha yako ya baadaye. Baada ya huu mwili kuisha huu hapa. Maisha yako ya baadaye yatakuwa wapi? Utakuwa umetengeneza maisha yako Mungu ata—akupe kibali, upate hiyo nafasi ya maisha ya baadaye. Mimi naona kitu kikubwa zaidi kuliko kutafuta mafamilia hapa ambayo yanapita.*

Chapter 4

EVANGELIST: *Aliende kwa waganga kabisa kwa sababu ya mke wake wakahangaika. Bahati nzuri walipokuja, kuna bwana mmoja anafanya KCMC. Tukamwambia hebu nenda muone yule wa KCMC akaende akampima na kumwambia kuwa mke wako anauvimbe kwenye kizazi*

> kwa namna hii si rahisi apate mtoto tena. Kwa namna hii tunakushauri . . . Huu uvimbe afanyiwe operation aondolewe na kizazi pia. Lakini yeye akasema huyu mke ninampenda sana ninaomba mnisaidie kumhudumia afanyiwe operation.

PASTOR: *Sasa yule mke wa kwanza alipoona upendo umepungua akamruhusu yule mume kwamba muoe huyu mwanamke. Ili asipigwe au chakula kiweze kuja nyumbani. Basi yule mwnaume akaenda akamuwoa yule hawara.*

PASTOR: *Sasa yule mke wa kwanza, Akasema na mchungaji ni mimi nilimruhusu. Kwahiyo sasa ukimwambia amfukuze huyu mdogo. . . [. . .] Ananiambia nimpeleke wapi, wote nawapenda, na ni mimi nilimponza. Yule mdogo yeye anasema wanijengee nyumba yangu mimi nitakwenda. Lakini mwanaume hana uwezo wa kujenga nyumba, Na alijua kwamba mume anampenda sana pia. Kwa hiyo ilikuwa ngumu sana. Yule mwana*
> *. . . nikabatiza watoto na mume akabakia alivyo.*

EVANGELIST: *Lakini katika kushirikiana hakunashida, hata wale watoto hawana shida, kwa hiyo walikuwa wanawaheshimu na wale watoto walikuwa na heshima.*

AULI: *Kwa hiyo hata watoto waliona kuwa ni mpango mzuri?*

EVANGELIST: *Ndiyo na hata kanisa ni kwamba liliwarudhisha kundini na halafu . . .*

AULI: *Wakakaa rasmi.*

EVANGELIST: *Ndiyo.*

AULI: *Sasa kwa mfano hawa ulio eleza ilikuwa hivi kwamba huyu mama wa kwanza alikaa peke yake au alipata watoto kutoka huyu mama mwingine ili amtunze unaonaje au aliishi peke yake?*

EVANGELIST: *Ni kwamba wale watoto wa mama mdogo wanamwona huyu kama ni mama sawa na yule mama yao.*

AULI: *Hivyo huyu mama mkubwa ni mama sawa?*

EVANGELIST: *Kwa hiyo hata kukaa wanaweza kuwa kokote tu.*

EVANGELIST: *Ni mwamba hata huyu aliyefariki mwezi uliopita, wale watoto walimfanyia heshima kubwa sana, kama ni jeneza, walibeba. . . . walimtunza vizuri tu, na hata yule mke mdogo alimheshimu tu.*

AULI: *Kwa hiyo hakuweza kumdhihaki kuwa hujapata mtoto.*

EVANGELIST: *Hapana haikuwa rahisi . . .*

UPENDO: *Hata hivyo nikimkuta mke wake, ninamwona kama ni mtu wa kawaida. Hakuna ugomvi wala nini . . .*

MRS: *Hana uwezo wa kuweza kujitegemea. Na siyo mama anayependa kufanya sana kazi za mikono. Anapenda kuuza vitu vidogo-vidogo kama vichungwa. [. . .] Sasa kidogo yeye ana watoto wengi kidogo. Na amezaa na watu tofauti. Lakini yeye kuzaa kwake ni ili aweze kupata uchumi, wakuweza yeye kupata mahitaji yake.*

PASTOR: *Haa! Upande mwingine kikanisa anatengwa! Lazima awekwe chini ya marudi. Kwa sababu kwa kweli alikwenda kinyume na ndoa yake. Kijamii, kifamilia, yule mtoto aliyezaliwa nje kama baba atasema ni wa kwake! Mila na desturi zitampa haki zote. Yule mtoto maana hana kosa. Na baba amesema ni wangu kwa sababu sikupata kuzaa kwa hiyo nimempata huyu, ni mtoto wangu. Ana haki ya kurithi. [. . .] Na katika familia hii baba akapata, akaenda kumtafuta wa kiume!*

Glossary

All words are in Swahili if not otherwise indicated.

Aibu	Shame
Bwanangu	A male partner
Hana nguvu za uume	He does not have the male capacity or power (refers to a childless man)
Hawara	A concubine, lover, or mistress
Heshima	Honor, respect, dignity
Kasoro	A defect, fault
Kienyeji	Traditional (in this study refers to the Chagga traditional beliefs and practices)
Kihamba	(Chagga) Permanently held inheritable banana garden in which coffee is also grown
Kikristo	Christian (in this study refers to the Christian heritage of the early missionaries)
Kimachame	The Machame dialect of the Chagga language, spoken in western Kilimanjaro
Kisasa	Modern (in this study refers to all modern things related to education, urbanization and modernization)
Kuoa	To marry (active, used for a man)
Kuolewa	To be married (passive, used for a woman)
Kuvumilia	To have patience or to tolerate
Laana	A curse
Mwanamke	A woman, not a respected wife in a community
Mke	A wife (an official term)

Mke mdogo	Literally, a second or younger wife (in common use means a concubine)
Mtu mzima	An adult (literally, a whole person)
Mume	A husband
Ndoa takatifu	Holy wedlock, marriage officiated in the church
Ndoa ya Mkristo	Marriage of a Christian
Siri	A secret, especially a family secret
Tasa	An infertile woman
Ujamaa	Tanzanian socialism during the time of President Nyerere
Uzima	Vitality, adulthood, completeness, existence, maturity, perfection
Volkskirche	(German) communal people's church (the missionary goal of the German Leipzig mission in Kilimanjaro)

Bibliography

Interview Material

INTERVIEWEES HAVE BEEN CODED in order to guarantee their anonymity. The first code element indicates the interview group category: "CW" refers to church worker, "P" to parishioner, and "CP" to childless person. The single digit that follows is a unique identifier. Sex is indicated by "f" (female) or "m" (male). The field research parish of the interviewee is identified by "U" for the urban parish, or "R" for the rural parish. The interview tapes and the transliterated texts are stored in my personal archives.

Church workers:

CW1m/U	13/10/2000
CW2m/U	13/10/2000
CW3m/U	14/10/2000
CW4m/U	25/10/2000
CW5f/U	25/10/2000
CW6f/U	8/12/2000
CW7f/U	5/2/2001
CW8m/U	6/2/2001
CW1m/R	5/12/2000
CW2m/R	12/1/2001
CW3m/R	12/1/2001 and 18/10/2001
CW4m/R	11/10/2001
CW5f/R	6/7/2001

Parishioners:

P1m/U	14/10/2000
P2f/U	14/10/2000 and 7/12/2001
P3f/U	24/10/2000
P4f/U	25/10/2000
P5f/U	25/10/2000
P6f/U	25/10/2000

Bibliography

P7f/U	25/10/2000
P8f/U	25/10/2000
P9f/U	8/12/2000
P10f/U	2/12/2001
P11f/U	23/11/2001
P12f/U	23/11/2001
P13f/U	1/3/2002
P1m/R	21/11/2000
P2f/R	21/11/2000
P3m/R	21/11/2000
P4f/R	21/11/2000
P5f/R and P6f/R	21/11/2000
P7m/R	18/10/2001

Childless persons:

CP1f/U	28/10/2000
CP2f/U	28/10/2000
CP1f/R	28/1/2001 FWD (and polygynous spouses)
CP2f/R	21/2/2001 FWD and 14/2/2002
CP3f/R	24/1/2001 FWD
CP3m/R	18/10/2001 FWD
CP4m/R	18/10/2001

Diary Material

Observations made during fieldwork, as well as four interviews, are recorded in the following fieldwork diaries, which are stored in my personal archives.

Fieldwork Diary 12/1999—2/2001, 80 pages
Fieldwork Diary 2/2001—3/2002, 80 pages
Fieldwork Diary (seminar notebook) 11/2000—2/2002, 58 pages

Literature

Albers, Robert H. *Shame: A Faith Perspective*. Binghamton, NY: Haworth, 1995.
Antonovsky, Aaron. *Health, Stress and Coping: New Perspectives on Mental and Physical Well-Being*. San Francisco: Jossey-Bass, 1979.
———. *Unraveling the Mystery of Health: How People Manage Stress and Stay Well*. San Francisco: Jossey-Bass, 1988.
Atkinson, Robert. *The Life Story Interview*. Qualitative Research Methods 44. Thousand Oaks, CA: Sage, 1998.

Bahemuka, Judith Mbula. "Social Changes and Women's Attitudes toward Marriage in East Africa." In *The Will to Arise: Women, Tradition, and the Church in Africa*, edited by Mercy Amba Oduyoye and Musimbi R. A. Kanyoro, 119–34. Maryknoll, NY: Orbis, 1992.

Bahemuka, Judith Mbula, and Joseph L. Brockington. Preface to *East Africa in Transition: Communities, Cultures, and Change*, edited by Judith M. Bahemuka and Joseph L. Brockington, xv–xvi. Nairobi: Acton, 2001.

Bahendwa, L. Festo. *Christian Religious Education in the Lutheran Dioceses of North-Western Tanzania*. Helsinki: Finnish Society for Missiology and Ecumenics, 1990.

Baumeister, Roy F., et al. "Interpersonal Aspects of Guilt: Evidence from Narrative Studies." In *Self-Conscious Emotions: The Psychology of Shame, Guilt, Embarrassment, and Pride*, edited by June Price Tangney and Kurt W. Fischer, 255–73. New York: Guilford, 1995.

Binau, Brad A. "Shame and the Human Predicament." In *Counseling and the Human Predicament: A Study of Sin, Guilt, and Forgiveness*, edited by LeRoy Aden and David G. Benner, 127–43. Grand Rapids: Baker, 1989.

———. "When Shame Is the Question, How Does the Atonement Answer?" *Journal of Pastoral Theology* 12, no. 1 (2002) 89–113.

Bülow, Dorthe von. "Power, Prestige and Respectability: Women's Groups in Kilimanjaro, Tanzania." Centre for Development Research Working Paper 95.11. Copenhagen: CDR, 1995.

Buthelezi, Manas. "Toward Indigenous Theology in South Africa." In *The Emergent Gospel: Theology from the Underside of History*, edited by Sergio Torres and Virginia Fabella, 56–75. Maryknoll, NY: Orbis, 1976.

Comaroff, Jean, and John Comaroff. *Revelation and Revolution: Christianity, Colonialism, and Consciousness in South Africa*. Vol. 1. Chicago: University of Chicago Press, 1991.

Domingues, Fernando. *Christ Our Healer: A Theological Reflection with Reference to Aylward Shorter*. Nairobi: Paulines Publications Africa, 2000.

Dundas, Charles. *Kilimanjaro and Its People: A History of the Wachagga, Their Laws, Customs and Legends*. London: Witherby, 1968 [1924].

Erikson, Erik H. *Identity, Youth, and Crisis*. New York: Norton, 1968.

Evangelical Lutheran Church in Tanzania. Constitution of the Evangelical Lutheran Church in Tanzania, Northern Diocese, 1986.

Finnegan, Ruth. *Oral Literature in Africa*. Oxford Library of African Literature. Nairobi: Oxford University Press, 1976.

Fleisch, Paul. *Lutheran Beginnings around Mt. Kilimanjaro: The first 40 Years*. Edited by Ernst Jaeschke. Usa River: Research Institute of Makumira University College, Tumaini University, 1998.

Flick, Uwe. *An Introduction to Qualitative Research*. Thousand Oaks, CA: Sage, 1998.

Folkman, Susan. "Personal Control and Stress and Coping Processes: A Theoretical Analysis." *Journal of Personality and Social Psychology* 46, no. 4 (1984) 839–52.

Folkman, Susan, and Richard S. Lazarus. "Coping and Emotion." In *Stress and Coping: An Anthology*, edited by Alan Monat and Richard S. Lazarus, 207–27. New York: Columbia University Press, 1991.

Frei, Hans W. *The Eclipse of Biblical Narrative: A Study of Eighteenth and Nineteenth Century Hermeneutics*. New Haven, MA: Yale University Press, 1974.

Freilich, Morris. "Toward a Formalization of Field Work." In *Marginal Natives: Anthropologists at Work*, edited by Morris Freilich et al., 485–585. New York: Harper & Row, 1970.
Georgakopoulou, Alexandra. "Thinking Big with Small Stories in Narrative and Identity Analysis." *Narrative Inquiry* 16, no. 1 (2006) 122–30.
Gijsels, Marjolein, et al. "'No Child Send' Context and Consequences of Female Infertility in North Western Tanzania." In *Women and Infertility in Sub-Saharan Africa: A Multi-disciplinary Perspective*, edited by J. Ties Boerma and Zaida Mgalla, 203–22. Amsterdam: Royal Tropical Institute, 2001.
Greil, Arthur, et al. "Infertility: His and Hers." *Gender & Society* 2, no. 2 (1988) 172–99.
Gutmann, Bruno. "Totenreich und Todesgedanken der Wadschagga." *Globus* 89 (1906) 197–200.
———. *Die Frau bei den Wadschagga*. Braundsohwei, Vieweg, 1907.
Haram, Liv. *"Women Out of Sight." Modern Women in Gendered Worlds: The Case of the Meru of Northern Tanzania*. Bergen: University of Bergen, 1999.
Harjula, Raimo. *God and Sun in Meru Thought*. Helsinki: Finnish Society for Missiology and Ecumenics, 1969.
———. *Syyllisyys, sairaus ja ihminen. Syyllisyys sairauden selityksenä eri kulttuureissa ja uskonnoissa*. Helsinki: Kirjapaja, 1986.
———. "Curse as a Manifestation of Broken Human Relationships among the Meru of Tanzania." In *Culture, Experience and Pluralism, Essays on African Ideas of Illness and Healing*, edited by Anita Jacobson-Widding and David Westerlund, 125–37. Uppsala Studies in Cultural Anthropology 13. Uppsala, Sweden: Uppsala University, 1989.
Hasu, Päivi. *Desire and Death: History through Ritual Practice in Kilimanjaro*. Transactions of the Finnish Anthropological Society 42. Helsinki: FAS, 1999.
Healey, Joseph, and Donald Sybertz. *Towards an African Narrative Theology*. Nairobi: Paulines Publications Africa, 1996.
Henin, Roushdi A. "Fertility, Infertility and Sub-fertility in Sub-Saharan Africa." Population Studies and Research Institute. Nairobi: University of Nairobi, 1982.
Hogg, Michael A., and Dominic Abrams. *Social Identifications: A Social Psychology of Intergroup Relations and Group Processes*. New York: Routledge, 1988.
Holstein, James A., and Jaber F. Gubrium. *The Self We Life By: Narrative Identity in a Postmodern World*. Oxford: Oxford University Press, 2000.
Howard, Mary Theresa, and Ann V. Millard. *Hunger and Shame: Child Malnutrition and Poverty on Mount Kilimanjaro*. New York: Routledge, 1997.
Inhorn, Marcia C. *Infertility and Patriarchy: The Cultural Politics of Gender and Family Life in Egypt*. Philadelphia: University of Pennsylvania Press, 1995.
Jacobson-Widding, Anita. *Chapungu: The Bird that Never Drops a Feather. Male and Female Identities in an African Society*. Uppsala Studies in Cultural Anthropology 28. Uppsala, Sweden: Uppsala University, 1999.
Järvikoski, Aila. "Sisäinen elämänhallinta ja sosiaaliset paineet." In *Elämänhallintaa etsimässä*, edited by Raimo Raitasalo, 35–45. Helsinki: Kansaneläkelaitos, 1996.
Jiwani, Shiraz. "The Use of Community-Level Data in the Analysis of Fertility Differentials in Tanzania." MA thesis, University of Dar es Salaam, 1976.
Kafunzile, Sylvester. "Shame and Its Effects among the Haya Women in North-Western Tanzania." PhD diss., Luther Seminary, 2001.
Kanyoro, Musimbi R. A. *Introducing Feminist Cultural Hermeneutics: An African Perspective*. New York: Sheffield Academic, 2002.

Kasonga wa Kasonga. "African Christian Palaver: A Contemporary Way of Healing Communal Conflicts and Crisis." In *The Church and Healing, Echoes from Africa*, edited by Emmanuel Lartey, Daisy Nwachuku, and Kasonga Wa Kasonga, 49–65. Frankfurt: Peter Lang, 1994.

Kaufman, Gershen. *The Psychology of Shame: Theory and Treatment of Shame-Based Syndromes*. New York: Springer, 1996.

Kayongo-Male Diane, and Philista Onyango. *The Sociology of the African Family*. New York: Longman, 1984.

Kerner, Donna O. "Chaptering the Narrative: The Material of Memory in Kilimanjaro, Tanzania." In *The Labyrinth of Memory: Ethnographic Journeys*, edited by Marea C. Teski and Jacob J. Climo, 113–27. Westport, CT: Bergin & Garvey, 1995.

Kielmann, Karina. "Barren Ground: Contesting Identities of Infertile Women in Pemba, Tanzania." In *Pragmatic Women and Body Politics*, edited by Margaret Lock and Patricia A. Kaufert, 127–63. Cambridge Studies in Medical Anthropology 5. Cambridge: Cambridge University Press, 1998.

Kvale, Steinar. *Interviews: An Introduction to Qualitative Research Interviewing*. Thousand Oaks, CA: Sage, 1996.

Kyomo, Andrew A. "Faith and Healing in the African Context." In *Charismatic Renewal in Africa: A Challenge for African Christianity*, edited by Mika Vähäkangas and Andrew A. Kyomo, 145–56. Nairobi: Acton, 2003.

Laitinen, Jorma. *Syntiinlankeemus, häpeä ja syyllisyys: Uskonnonfilosofinen tutkielma*. Helsinki: Suomalainen Teologinen Kirjallisuusseura, 2002.

Larrain, Jorge. *Ideology & Cultural Identity: Modernity and the Third World Presence*. Cambridge: Polity, 1994.

Larsen, Ulla, and Han Raggers. "Levels and Trends in Infertility in Sub-Saharan Africa." In *Women and Infertility in Sub-Saharan Africa: A Multi-disciplinary Perspective*, edited by J. Ties Boerma and Zaida Mgalla, 26–69. Amsterdam: Royal Tropical Institute, 2001.

Larsson, Birgitta. *Conversion to Greater Freedom?: Women, Church and Social Change in North Western Tanzania under Colonial Rule*. Studia Historica Upsaliensia 162. Uppsala, Sweden: Uppsala University, 1991.

Lawuo, Z. E. *Education and Social Change in a Rural Community. A Study of Colonial Education and Local Response among the Chagga between 1920 and 1945*. Dar es Salaam: Dar es Salaam University Press, n.d.

Lieblich, Amia, et al. *Narrative Research: Reading, Analysis and Interpretation*. Applied Social Research Methods Series 47. Thousand Oaks, CA: Sage, 1998.

Lindbeck, George A. *The Nature of Doctrine: Religion and Theology in a Postliberal Age*. London: SPCK, 1984.

Linde, Charlotte. *Life Stories: The Creation of Coherence*. New York: Oxford University Press, 1993.

Longman, Tremper, III. *Literary Approaches to Biblical Interpretation*. Foundations of Contemporary Interpretation 3. Grand Rapids: Academie Books, Zondervan, 1987.

Lugazia, Faith J. "Charismatic Movements and the Evangelical Lutheran Church in Tanzania." In *Charismatic Renewal in Africa: A Challenge for African Christianity*, edited by Mika Vähäkangas and Andrew A. Kyomo, 45–65. Nairobi: Acton, 2003.

Malewo, Jackson A. "Pastoral Counselling." In *The Ministry of Healing*, 80–102. Staff Institute of ATIEA: Addis Ababa, 1990.

———. *Pre-marital Counseling in the Parish: Preventing Future Marital Problems in Families*. Makumira Publication 8. Erlangen, Ger.: Erlanger Verlag für Mission und Ökumene, 2002.

Malle, Anastasia. "Hagar Names God: A Woman's Vision Arising in the Midst of Pain, Genesis 16 and 21." M.Th. thesis, Wartburg Theological Seminary, 1992.

———. "Interpreting the Lament Psalms from the Tanzanian Context: Problems and Prospects." Ph.D. diss, Luther Seminary, 2000.

Mann, Chris. "Family Fables," in *Narrative and Genre*, edited by Mary Chamberlain and Paul Thomson, 81–98. New York: Routledge, 1998.

Marealle, Petro Itosi. *Maisha ya Mchagga hapa duniani*. N.p, 1947.

Masamba ma Mpolo, Jean. "Spirituality and Counselling for Healing and Liberation: The Context and Praxis of African Pastoral Activity and Psychotherapy." In *The Church and Healing, Echoes from Africa*, edited by Emmanuel Lartey, Daisy Nwachuku, and Kasonga Wa Kasonga, 11–34. Frankfurt: Peter Lang, 1994.

Matta, Overa. "Church Discipline: It's Bases and Practice in the Evangelical Lutheran Church in Tanzania, Northern Diocese." BD research paper, Makumira University College, Tumaini University, 1989.

Mbiti, John S. *African Religions & Philosophy*. Nairobi: Heinemann, 1969.

———. *Love and Marriage in Africa*. London: Longman, 1973.

McClendon, James William. *Biography as Theology: How Life Stories Can Remake Today's Theology*. Nashville: Abingdon, 1974.

McGuire, Meredith B. *Religion, the Social Context*. Belmond, CA: Wadsworth, 1997.

McIntyre, Alasdair. *After Virtue: A Study in Moral Theory*. Notre Dame: University of Notre Dame Press, 1981.

Mgalla, Zaida and Ties Boerma. "The Discourse of Infertility in Tanzania." In *Women and Infertility in Sub-Saharan Africa: A Multi-disciplinary Perspective*, edited by J. Ties Boerma and Zaida Mgalla, 190–200. Amsterdam: Royal Tropical Institute, 2001.

Miall, Charlene E. "The Stigma of Involuntary Childlessness." *Social Problems* 33, no. 4 (1986) 267–82.

Mitchell, W. T., editor. *On Narrative*. Chicago: Chicago University Press, 1981.

Mndeme, Mathias Gerson. "Healing Ministry in the Church in Tanzania." D.Min. thesis, Trinity Lutheran Seminary, 1982.

Moore, Sally Falk. "Selection for Failure in a Small Social Field: Ritual Concord and Fraternal Strife: Kilimanjaro 1968–69." In *Symbol and Politics in Communal Ideology: Cases and Questions*, edited by Sally Falk Moore and Barbara G. Myerhoff, 109–43. Symbol, Myth, and Ritual Series. Ithaca: Cornell University Press, 1975.

———. "The Secret of the Men." *Africa* 46, no. 4, (1976) 357–69.

———. "The Chagga of Kilimanjaro." In *The Chagga and Meru of Tanzania*, by Sally Falk Moore and Paul Puritt, edited by William M. O'Bar. Ethnographic Survey of Africa, East Central Africa, 18. London: International African Institute, 1977.

———. *Social Facts and Fabrications: "Customary" Law on Kilimanjaro, 1880–1980*. Lewis Henry Morgan Lectures, 1981. Cambridge: Cambridge University Press, 1986.

Mosha, Raymond Sambuli. *The Heartbeat of Indegenous Africa: A Study of the Chagga Educational System*. Garland Reference Library of Social Science, Indigenous Knowledge and Schooling 3. New York: Garland, 2000.

Mtenga, C. B. "The Value of Children and Fertility in Kilimanjaro Region: A Case Study of Mwanga District." MA thesis, University of Dar es Salaam, 1994.

Munga, Anneth Nyagawa. "The Understanding and Practice of Church Discipline in the Evangelical Lutheran Church in Tanzania, North Eastern Diocese." BD research paper, Makumira University College, Tumaini University, 1989.

———. *Uamsho: A Theological Study of the Proclamation of the Revival Movement within the Evangelical Lutheran Church in Tanzania*. Studia Theologica Lundensia 54. Lund, Sweden: Lund University Press, 1998.

Nasimiyu-Wasike, Anne. "Polygamy, A Feminist Critique." In *The Will to Arise: Women, Tradition, and the Church in Africa*, edited by Mercy Amba Oduyoye and Musimbi R. A. Kanyoro, 101–18. Maryknoll, NY: Orbis, 1995.

Navone, John. *Seeking God in Story*. Collegeville, MN: Liturgical, 1990.

Ngallaba, Sylvester A. M. M. "Fertility Differentials in Tanzania with Special Reference to Four Regions." MA thesis, University of Dar es Salaam, 1972.

Ngavatula, Alphonce Msemwa. "The Concept of Adumile (Menopause) among the Bena in Relation to Christian Marriage: A Case Study in the ELCT: Southern Diocese." BD research paper, Makumira University College, Tumaini University, 2002.

Njoroge, Nyambura J. "Groaning and Languishing in Labour Pains." In *Groaning in Faith: African Women in the Household of God*, edited by Musimbi R. A. Kanyoro and Nyambura J. Njoroge, 3–15. Nairobi: Acton, 1996.

Njuu, S. "Traditional Marriage among the Chagga." Occasional Reseach Paper 252, Makerere University, 1974.

Nwachuku, Daisy N. "Perceptions on Family Counselling in Present Nigeria." In *Pastoral Care and Counselling in Africa Today*, edited by Jean Masamba ma Mpolo and Daisy Nwachuku, 100–114. African Pastoral Studies 1. Frankfurt: Peter Lang, 1991.

———. "Rituals and Symbols in the Healing of Infertility in Africa: Pastoral Counselling Response." In *The Church and Healing, Echoes from Africa*, edited by Emmanuel Lartey, Daisy Nwachuku, and Kasonga Wa Kasonga, 66–84. Frankfurt: Peter Lang, 1994.

Oduyoye, Mercy Amba. "A Critique of Mbiti's View on Love and Marriage in Africa." In *Religious Plurality in Africa: Essays in Honour of John S. Mbiti*, edited by Jacob K. Olupona and Sulayman S. Nyang, 341–65. Religion and Society 32. Berlin: de Gruyter, 1993.

———. "Feminist Theology in an African Perspective." In *Paths of African Theology*, edited by Rosino Gibellini, 166–81. London: SCM, 1994.

Okpewho, Isidore. *The Epic in Africa: Toward a Poetics of the Oral Performance*. New York: Columbia University Press, 1979.

Omari, Cuthbert K. "Fertility Rates and the Status of Women in Tanzania." In *Gender, Family, and Household in Tanzania*, edited by Colin Greighton and C. K. Omari, 253–68. Brookfield, VT: Avebury, 1995.

Orobaton, Nosa. "Dimensions of Sexuality among Nigerian Men: Perspectives for Fertility." In *Fertility and the Male Life-Cycle in the Era of Fertility Decline*, edited by Caroline Bledsoe et al., 207–30. International Studies in Demography. New York: Oxford University Press, 2000.

Parrinder, E. Geoffrey. *African Traditional Religion*. 3rd ed. London: Sheldon, 1974.

Peil, Margaret, and Olatunji Oyeneve. *Consensus, Conflict and Change: A Sociological Introduction to African Societies*. Nairobi: East African Educational Pub., 1998.

Pietilä, Tuulikki. *Gossip, Markets and Gender: The Dialogical Construction of Morality in Kilimanjaro*. Helsingin yliopiston Sosiologian laitoksen tutkimuksia 233. Helsinki: Dept. of Social Anthropology, University of Helsinki, 1999.

Pike, Kenneth L. *Language in Relation to a Unified Theory of the Structure of Human Behaviour.* Janua Linguarum, Series Maior 24. The Hague: Mouton, 1971.

Pobee, John S. "Life and Peace: An African Perspective." In *Variations in Christian Theology in Africa,* edited by Carl Hallencreutz and John Pobee, 14–31. Nairobi: Uzima, 1986.

Polkinghorne, Donald. "Narrative Configuration in Qualitative Analysis." In *Life History and Narrative,* edited by J. Amos Hatch and Richard Wisniewski, 5–24. Washington, DC: Falmer, 1995.

Raitasalo, Raimo "Aaron Antonoskyn salutogeeninen malli ja elämänhallinta." In *Elämänhallintaa etsimässä,* edited by Raimo Raitasalo, 57–76. Helsinki: Kansaneläkelaitos, 1996.

Raum, Otto Friedrich. *Chaga Childhood: A Description of Indigenous Education in an East African Tribe.* New introduction by Sally Falk Moore. Classics in African Anthropology. Hamburg: International African Institute and LIT, 1996 [1940].

Ricoeur, Paul. *Time and Narrative.* Translated by Kathleen McLaughlin and David Pellauer. 3 vols. Chicago: University of Chicago Press, 1984–88.

———. *Oneself as Another.* Translated by Kathleen Blamey. Chicago: University of Chicago Press, 1992.

Riessman, Catherine Kohler. *Narrative Analysis.* Qualitative Research Methods 30. Newbury Park, CA: Sage, 1993.

———. "Even If We Don't Have Children (We) Can Live: Stigma and Infertility in South India." In *Narrative and the Cultural Construction of Illness and Healing,* edited by Cheryl Mattingly and Linda C. Garro, 128–52. Berkeley: University of California Press, 2000.

———. "Personal Troubles as Social Issues: A Narrative of Infertility in Context." In *Qualitative Research in Social Work,* edited by Ian F. Shaw and Nick G. Gould, 73–82. Introducing Qualitative Methods. Thousand Oaks, CA: Sage, 2001.

Riihinen, Olavi. "Elämänhallinta-käsitteen erittelyä ja ongelmia." In *Elämänhallintaa etsimässä,* edited by Raimo Raitasalo, 16–33. Helsinki: Kansaneläkelaitos, 1996.

Riwa, Peter N. M. "The Effect of Sex Preference for Children on Fertility: A Case Study from Two Villages in Moshi Rural District in Tanzania." MA thesis, University of Dar es Salaam, 1987.

Scheff, Thomas J. "Conflict in Family Systems: The Role of Shame." In *Self-Conscious Emotions: The Psychology of Shame, Guilt, Embarrassment, and Pride,* edited by June Price Tangney and Kurt W. Fischer, 393–412. New York: Guilford, 1995.

Schoepf, Brooke Grundfest. "Inscribing the Body Politic: Women and AIDS in Africa." In *Pragmatic Women and Body Politics,* edited by Margaret Lock and Patricia A. Kaufert, 98–126. Cambridge: Cambridge University Press, 1998.

Setel, Philip. "The Social Context of AIDS Education among Young Men in Northern Kilimanjaro." In *Young People at Risk" Fighting AIDS in Northern Tanzania,* edited by Knut-Inge Kepp, Paul M. Biswalo, and Aud Talle, 49–68. Oslo: Scandinavian University Press, 1995.

Setel, Philip et. al. "Men's Perspectives on Fertility and Fatherhood in Urban Kilimanjaro." Health Transition Working Paper 25. Health Transition Centre, National Institute for Epidemiology and Population Health, Australian National University, 1997.

Shao, Martin F. *Bruno Gutmann's Missionary Method and its Influence on the Evangelical Lutheran Church in Tanzania Northern Diocese.* World Mission Scripts 2. Erlangen: Erlanger Verlag für Mission und Ökumene, 1990.

Shoo, Fredrick O. "Tanzania: Church in a Changing Society." Diss., Augustana Hochschule, Germany, 1995.
Shoo, Kaleb. "Traditional African Marriage among the Chagga-Mashami in Relation to Christian Marriage." Diploma research paper, Makumira University College, Tumaini University, 1979.
Shorter, Aylward. *African Culture, an Overview: Social-Cultural Anthropology.* Nairobi: Paulines Publications Africa, 1998.
Silberschmidt, Margrethe. *"Women Forget that Men are the Masters": Gender Antagonism and Socio-Economic Change in Kisii District, Kenya.* Uppsala, Sweden: Nordiska Afrikainstitutet, 1999.
Sintonen, Teppo. *Etninen identiteetti ja narratiivisuus, Kanadan suomalaiset miehet elämänsä kertojina.* Jyväskylä, Finland: University of Jyväskylä, 1999.
Smedjebacka, Henrik. *Lutheran Church Autonomy in Northern Tanzania, 1940–1963.* Åbo (Turku), Finland: Åbo Akademi, 1973.
Spradley, James P. *Participant Observation.* New York: Holt, Rinehart and Winston, 1980.
Stahl, Kathleen M. *History of the Chagga People of Kilimanjaro.* Studies in African History, Anthropology and Ethnology 2. The Hague: Mouton, 1964.
Stambach, Amy. *Lessons from Mount Kilimanjaro: Schooling, Community, and Gender in East Africa.* New York: Routledge, 2000.
Stiver, Dan R. *The Philosophy of Religious Language: Sign, Symbol, and Story.* Oxford: Blackwell, 1996.
Svartvik, Jasper. *Mark and Mission: Mk 7: 1–23 in Its Narrative and Historical Contexts.* Coniectanea biblica, New Testament Series 32. Stockholm: Almqvist & Wiksell, 2000.
Swai, Wilbard. "Christian Marriage Counselling: A Case Study in ELCT—Northern Diocese, Hai Eastern District." BD research paper, Makumira University College, Tumaini University, 2002.
Swantz, Marja-Liisa. *The Religious and Magical Rites Connected with the Life Cycle of the Woman in Some Bantu Ethnic Groups in Tanzania.* Dar es Salaam: n.p., 1966.
———. *Women in Development: A Creative Role Denied? The Case of Tanzania.* London: C. Hurst, 1985.
Tangney, June Price. "Shame and Guilt in Interpersonal Relationships." In *Self-Conscious Emotions: The Psychology of Shame, Guilt, Embarrassment, and Pride,* edited by June Price Tangney and Kurt W. Fischer, 114–39. New York: Guilford, 1995.
———. "Hai District: Total Population by Age in Single Years, Five-Year Age Groups and Sex." *2002 Population and Housing Census* Web site. Online: http://www.tanzania.go.tz/census/districts/hai.htm.
Tanzania Parliament. *Law of Marriage Act, 1971.* Act 5/71. Jamhuri ya Muungano wa Tanzania, 1971.
Taylor, Steven J., and Robert Bogdan. *Introduction to Qualitative Research Methods: The Search for Meanings.* New York: Wiley, 1984.
Tempels, Placide. *La philosophie bantoue.* Translated from Dutch by A. Rubbens. Elisabethville, Congo: Lovania, 1945.
Terry, Deborah J., et al. "Attitude-Behaviour Relations: Social Identity and Group Membership." In *Attitudes, Behavior, and Social Context: The Role of Norms and Group Membership,* edited by Deborah J. Terry and Michael A. Hogg, 67–93. Mahwah, NJ: L. Erlbaum, 2000.
Tessler, Mark A., et al. *Tradition and Identity in Changing Africa.* New York: Harper & Row, 1973.

Townsend, Nicholas W. "Male Fertility as a Lifetime of Relationships: Contextualizing Men's Biological Reproduction in Botswana." *Fertility and the Male Life-Cycle in the Era of Fertility Decline*, edited by Caroline Bledsoe et al., 343–64. International Studies in Demography. New York: Oxford University Press, 2000.

Trafimow, David. "A Theory of Attitudes, Subjective Norms, and Private versus Collective Self-Concepts." In *Attitudes, Behavior, and Social Context: The Role of Norms and Group Membership*, edited by Deborah J. Terry and Michael A. Hogg, 47–65. Mahwah, NJ: L. Erlbaum, 2000.

Turner, John C. Foreword in *Social Identifications: A Social Psychology of Intergroup Relations and Group Processes*, by Michael Hogg and Dominic Abrams, x–xii. New York: Routledge, 1988.

Uka, E. M. "The African Family and Issues of Women's Infertility." *Africa Theological Journal*, 20, no. 3 (1991) 189–200.

Urio, Aaron. *The Concept of Memory in the Chagga Life Cycle in Relation to Christian Eucharistic Traditions*. Erlangen, Ger.: Erlanger Verlag für Mission und Ökumene, 1990.

Vähäkangas, Auli. "Responses to Prayer Healing in the ELCT Northern Diocese." In *Charismatic Renewal in Africa: A Challenge for African Christianity*, edited by Mika Vähäkangas and Andrew A. Kyomo, 157–68. Nairobi: Acton, 2003.

Vähäkangas, Mika. "Ukristo, Uzima, na Ujamaa: The Theology of the Evangelical Lutheran Church in Tanzania in Relation to Tanzanian Socialism." M.Th. thesis, University of Helsinki, 1992.

Vuorela, Ulla. *The Women's Question and the Modes of Human Reproduction: An Analysis of a Tanzanian Village*. Transactions of the Finnish Anthropological Society 20. Helsinki: Finnish Society for Development Studies, 1987.

Wallbott, Harald G., and Klaus R. Scherer. "Cultural Determinants in Experiencing Shame and Guilt." In *Self-Conscious Emotions: The Psychology of Shame, Guilt, Embarrassment, and Pride*, edited by June Price Tangney and Kurt W. Fischer, 465–87. New York: Guilford, 1995.

Waruta Douglas W. "Marriage and Family in Contemporary African Society." In *Pastoral Care in African Christianity: Challenging Essays in Pastoral Theology*, edited by Douglas W. Waruta and Hannah W. Kinoti, 101–19. Nairobi: Acton, 2000.

Welbourn, F. B. "Some Problems of African Christianity: Guilt and Shame." In *Christianity in Tropical Africa: Studies Presented and Discussed at the Seventh International African Seminar, University of Ghana, April 1965*, edited by C. G. Baëta, 182–96. London: International African Institute/Oxford University Press, 1968.

Westerlund, David. "Marriage and Religion: A Study of the Parliamentary Debates on the Marriage Bill in Tanzania 1971." *Temenos* 15 (1979) 96–113.

Index

Abrams, Dominic, 112–14
adoption, 47, 64–70, 140–41, 145, 160
Albers, Robert, 126–28, 133–37, 146–47, 156
Antonovsky, Aaron, 138–49, 152

Binau, Brad, 126–28, 133–35, 154–55

Chagga culture, 34, 74–75, 77, 87, 108, 115, 118, 124, 127, 129, 133, 139
Chagga family, 4–5, 11, 76, 100, 127, 129, 140, 146
childlessness, 9–10, 13, 17, 21, 27, 30, 43–44, 54, 61, 65–66, 70, 86, 108, 111, 113, 119, 126, 131–34, 137, 139, 146–48, 155
Christian marriage, 2–9, 17–21, 47, 69–70, 74, 78, 90, 99, 105–7, 147–48, 156–57
church discipline, 6–8, 48, 57, 79–82, 90–93, 97, 102–8, 117, 124, 134, 141, 146, 154
coping, 47, 56, 65, 70, 78–79, 83, 109, 111, 132, 137–48, 149–57, 160
cultural categories, 4–5, 21, 92, 89–93, 113–16, 120–23, 139, 147–48, 150–60
curse, 17, 131–32, 156, 173

desertion, 48, 50, 73–93, 102–5
divorce, 7, 9–10, 17, 48, 56–57, 77–79, 91, 99–101, 108–9

ELCT, 5–6, 107

family interference, 15, 19–20, 47, 57, 73, 90, 140
family secrets, 38, 47, 83, 127, 142, 160
female identity, 11, 14, 91, 120–25
fertility, 2, 9–10, 12–15, 38, 116, 123

gospel and culture, 116, 151
guilt, 47, 78, 125–32, 135, 141, 156

Hasu, Päivi, 11–12, 90, 107, 161
HIV/AIDS, 3, 8, 11–12, 89–90, 105, 140
healing, 78, 80, 155–57
Hogg, Michael, 112–14
honor, 82, 133–35, 141

immortality, 2, 10, 19, 31, 66, 75–76, 89, 152–55, 160
infertility, 2, –3, 9–16, 19, 21, 60–65, 69–70, 71–73, 88–89, 94–95, 104, 109–10
inheritance, 47, 67, 84, 88, 102, 119, 131
Inhorn, Marcia, 14–15, 70, 77
insults, 47, 57–60, 69, 128–132

Kilimanjaro area, 1, 3–9, 11–13, 23, 54, 65, 89, 131

male identity, 14, 68, 86, 92, 116–20, 123–24, 135, 161

Index

Machame, 4–5, 11, 19, 23–25, 35–36, 56–57, 65, 84, 113–16, 131, 153
model narratives, 42–43, 49–53, 113, 117, 122, 136, 145, 149, 155, 157–58
modern values, 89–93, 124
Malewo, Jackson, 18–19, 69, 157
Moore, Sally Falk, 10, 131

narrative analysis, 37–40, 45, 50–54
narrative theory, 41–44
Northern Diocese, 5–9, 17–19, 23, 74–75, 79–80, 94–95, 107–10, 115–16, 119, 124, 141, 147–48, 152

Oduyoye, Mercy Amba, 130, 153–54
oral tradition, 37–39

pastoral problem, 33, 97, 107–10, 119
patriarchal, 57–58, 61, 67, 74–76, 90, 113, 122–35, 145
personal identity, 5, 43, 111–13, 156, 158
polygyny, 8, 17, 47–48, 77, 94–110, 118, 136, 145, 152

Riessman, Catherine Kohler, 15, 42, 45, 52
rural, 1–5, 12, 14, 24–25, 34, 46–48, 69, 76, 80, 89–93, 104–8, 114, 118, 124, 129, 133, 145

sense of coherence, 139, 143, 146, 149–52, 155–57
Setel, Philip, 12, 109, 120
shame, 20, 47, 80, 125–37, 141–42, 154–56, 159–60
social change, 2–4, 21, 89–90, 144
social identity, 68, 77, 91–92, 103, 112–16, 122–25, 147, 150, 156, 159
stigma, 2, 44, 67, 70, 86, 89, 91, 119, 121, 132, 134, 136, 149, 159

tension management, 137–47, 159–60
traditional values, 18, 48, 89–93, 118, 145–47

urban, 1–5, 14, 21, 24–25, 34–35, 46, 48, 57–58, 69, 86, 89–90, 104, 106–8, 114, 117–18, 124, 135, 140, 159, 160–61
Urio, Aaron, 19, 66, 115–16, 151–53

wholeness, 73, 148–57

www.ingramcontent.com/pod-product-compliance
Lightning Source LLC
Chambersburg PA
CBHW062044220426
43662CB00010B/1644